Increasing Childhood Diseases & Developmental Disorders

VACCeptable Injuries?

Revealing Information

Markus Heinze

A LITERATURE REVIEW AND COLLECTION OF PERSONAL STORIES OF THE HARM VACCINES DO TO OUR CHILDREN

As a parent, for your child

Disclaimer

I am not a doctor, and I have never been a health-care professional of any kind. I am a concerned father of two beautiful children. I am not providing medical advice, nor am I telling parents not to vaccinate their children. I am simply sharing my discoveries with you. The decision on whether to vaccinate your children is entirely left up to you. I hope the information this book provides will help you to make an informed decision.

About the Author

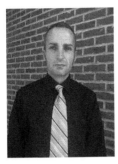 My name is Markus Heinze. I am originally from Germany. I came to America as a twenty-three-year-old to volunteer in Harlan County, KY. I taught at a small Catholic private school, and during the summers, I repaired houses. I went to school in Germany and the United States. I received an MA in Secondary Education from Union College and a BA in Psychology from Northern Kentucky University. I hold a teaching certificate in Kentucky and Ohio. I have taught German and French at Holy Trinity School in Harlan, KY; German at Bayer Corporation in Cincinnati, OH; Lakota Local Schools in West Chester, OH; Madison Local Schools in Middletown, OH; Oak Hills Local Schools in Cincinnati, OH and am currently employed by Cincinnati Public Schools in Cincinnati, Ohio. This is my fifteenth year of teaching. Most importantly, though, I am the husband of a wonderful wife (an elementary teacher) and the father of two beautiful and intelligent children.

Table of Contents

1. Introduction 6

2. The Reason for My Journey 12

3. The Known and Unknown 18

4. Challenging Information 22

5. Vaccine Controversy 28

6. Do Vaccines Work? 34

7. Funny, Yet Serious... 40

8. Did Diseases Decline Because of Vaccines? 42

9. Are Vaccines Safe? 46

10. Various Vaccines and The Damage They Cause............ 52

11. Scientifically Wrong Vaccine Safety Studies 58

12. Dr. Maurice Hilleman versus Your Pediatrician—
    A Comparison 64

13. Strong Opposition – Why Vaccines are Promoted 68

14. Credibility Issues 74

15. Pediatricians, Vaccines, and the Hippocratic Oath 78

16. Vaccine Research and Confirmation Bias 82

17. Doctors Who Left the Bandwagon 86

18. Something Personal or What's at Stake........................ 90

19. Vaccines Turning Our World Upside Down 94

20. Diabetes Mellitus and Vaccines.....................98

21. Our Daughter and Type-1 Diabetes 100

22. New Reality 106

23. Johanna and Multiple Vaccines –
    From Insult to Injury..112

24. More About the Hepatitis B Vaccine 116

25. Correlation versus Causality 120

26. Molecular Mimicry 122

27. Does an Autoimmune Vaccine Cause an Autoimmune
    Disease? 124

28. The End 126

29. End Notes 132

30. (End Notes) 142

Introduction

You are about to become a parent. Inside your womb, a little miracle is growing. If you are like my wife and I, you take a proactive approach to your child's safety. You find the best car seats, the safest toys, plan your child's educational future. Basically you are looking at everything and anything; after all, you want nothing but the best for your unborn child.

The moment arrives. As you are holding your newborn child in your arms for the first time, someone in the next room or down the hall prepares a little shot for your baby. Soon your baby will be injected with neurotoxins and other preservatives, and its immune system will be challenged to its core. This is one aspect you haven't researched, as you haven't heard about anyone *not* jumping on the vaccination bandwagon.

You wouldn't take a chance on car seats, on formula, cribs, or toys, but you are unknowingly taking one on vaccines. If you're lucky, you'll take your child home soon. If you aren't lucky, you may experience what other parents in your situation have experienced: a vaccine-injured child. Now, as you are aware of not having researched vaccines you become proactive. This book will help guide you making an informed decision.

Every year, tens of thousands of children in America and around the world are severely injured or killed by vaccines. This isn't an urban myth or a debatable accusation—it's an easily verifiable fact; the US government keeps a database recording such events. Nonetheless, the vast majority of people have no idea that vaccines pose both obvious and hidden dangers to their children—until their own child experiences a severe vaccine-related reaction.

You don't have to play the lottery with your children's life, hoping nothing goes wrong when they are injected with the potentially lethal neurotoxins routinely included in vaccines. This book provides you with a review of the medical and scientific literature surrounding vaccination risks as well as personal stories from those whose lives have been touched by vaccine-related injuries. My goal is to make you a better-informed parent. Given the information in this book, you hopefully will not have to experience what other parents have experienced: taking a healthy son or daughter in for immunizations and returning home with a severely disabled, sick, or dead child.

Medical interventions are difficult decisions, especially when parents have to make these decisions for their little children. Having to choose whether or not to intervene medically is simple if your child is ill and the medical intervention has proven to make your child feel better. If your child is healthy, however, the decision to medically intervene becomes more difficult, especially when the information on the effectiveness on the medical intervention is conflicting and inconclusive. Vaccinating your child is one of those medical interventions. Unfortunately most parents don't even realize that they are making a decision, as they follow blindly the recommendation of their pediatrician. Only parents whose children have been harmed by a vaccine, or who know children who have been harmed by a vaccine, tend to research the topic of vaccine safety and effectiveness on their own. I am one of those parents.

My teachers always told me that there was nothing worse than following blindly, as in doing so, I was empowering a group of a few to make decisions for the masses. Some of my teachers had seen Nazism and Stalinism and knew very well what they were talking about. There are great dangers involved in riding any bandwagon. Once we parents take our seats on the bandwagon, we are not longer leading our families—we are simply fellow passengers along with our children. We are no longer the ones making decisions for ourselves or our kids—we have ceded this important responsibility to whomever is driving that particular bandwagon. And this is a mistake. In any wagonload of people, the needs of individual passengers may differ greatly, and what might be good for the majority of the passengers might be quite dangerous—even deadly—for one or two of them. And if one of those two is our child, it is our responsibility—not the driver's—to foresee the danger and keep her from taking that deadly trip.

Whether or not you decide to vaccinate, hopefully this book will help you make an informed choice, rather than a bandwagon decision.

Unfortunately, the precautions I took didn't prevent the harm done to our daughter. Writing this book was a personal journey for me—a journey to discover what caused my daughter to develop type-1 diabetes. In her case, I believe that the hepatitis B vaccine after birth triggered an unstoppable reaction. In the course of my research, however, I've become convinced that *all* vaccines have the potential to cause children harm.

Even so, I wasn't quite sure whether or not I should publish this work. After all, I am not trying to get anyone to climb onto a bandwagon of my own. I don't have any simple answers to offer; certainly, I don't believe that the whole pharmaceutical industry and all of its products are all bad—in fact, sometimes, I find that they're extremely helpful. When our kids are sick, my wife and I don't use homeopathic medicine. We don't put nettle leaves on our son's ears when he gets an ear infection—he gets antibiotics. And he uses tubes as well, because tubes have been shown to be an effective treatment. When our children have fevers, we give them medicine that helps make them comfortable, as research has shown for these medicines to be effective.

In other words, I'm simply a rational person who looks at the available research in order to make medical decisions for my children. If you've picked up this book and read this far, you're probably the same sort of person— you love your children, and you want to know what the available research says about vaccinations. You realize that asking questions is an important point of being a responsible parent.

And that's why I finally decided that I needed to publish this book. Knowing what I know now about the dangers posed by vaccines, it would be extremely irresponsible of me to not share what I've learned.

Some will try to discredit my work by arguing that I am not a doctor, but I have been engaged long enough in scientific research and thought to consider myself an independent scientist. I would argue that I have done more independent research on the issue of vaccine effectiveness and safety than the average pediatrician. I hold a BA in Psychology and an MA in Education. I understand the Scientific Method, the rules of logic, and I know how to perform academic research. As such, I am more than qualified to find, read, and understand scientific research studies, and to realize that they clearly show that vaccines are a danger to our children. Those of us who have researched, and perhaps personally experienced the harm that vaccines can cause are motivated to speak out on this issue solely from a concern for the well-being of children. We have no conflict of interest.

The Reason for My Journey

On September 28, 2011, my three-year-old daughter, Johanna, was diagnosed with type-1 diabetes, an auto-immune disorder. As there's no history of type-1 diabetes in my or my wife's immediate family, we couldn't establish a genetic link, leading us to look for external factors. At Johanna's diagnosis, an A1C test was performed, measuring her glucose levels over the past three months. When comparing the A1C results to the onset of symptoms as expressed by behavioral signs, it became evident that the onset of Johanna's autoimmune disorder and the administration of vaccines matched.

I have been screened for positive autoantibodies, and none were found. My wife has been screened for positive autoantibodies, and none were found—neither of us passed diabetes on to our daughter. My parents have no signs of type-1 diabetes, and neither did my grandparents. I have four brothers and sisters; none have type-1 diabetes. My wife's parents have no signs of type-1 diabetes, and neither does her brother. Her grandparents never showed signs of type-1 diabetes.

There's no genetic link; therefore something must have overcome Johanna's natural resistance to type-1 diabetes. Numerous medical articles suggest that vaccine adjuvants (by definition, an adjuvant is an ingredient intended to aid in the effectiveness of the vaccine, substances such as aluminum and mercury) can cause autoimmune disorders. Shaw Tomljenovic, from the *National Center for Biotechnology Information* states:

"experimental evidence shows that simultaneous administration of as little as two to three immune adjuvants can overcome genetic resistance to autoimmunity."[1]

Vaccines caused my daughter to develop an autoimmune disorder—possibly for the rest of her life. And they have no doubt caused other children to suffer from type-1 diabetes and other autoimmune disorders. Research shows that when one part of the immune system is overexcited, the others may not function adequately, and the one targeted is likely to react excessively and ineffectively, such as in the case of allergies and autoimmune disease.

Whenever Johanna was vaccinated, signs of allergies appeared. We could never quite figure out why she would have allergies in the middle of winter. The signs of allergies disappeared a few weeks after the vaccines were administered, but now she suffers from an autoimmune disease. Why? Because her immune system reacted excessively and ineffectively to the vaccines she was given.

My research journey took me to Germany, Israel, and the US. The deeper that journey led me into vaccine safety, the more emotional this research became as I realized that I had needlessly harmed my child by having her vaccinated. I found pediatricians, general practitioners, and scientists falling victim to confirmation bias—only looking for, or only accepting, research that supported their pro-vaccine arguments. As I have listened to many of the pro-vaccine arguments given by pediatricians to persuade concerned parents, I was astonished that a simple search at the National Library of Medicine provided me with an abundance of credible research articles showing the harm vaccines can do.

In a research article conducted by the *Department of Medicine at the Ottawa Hospital Research Institute*, the researchers concluded, "There are significantly elevated risks of primarily emergency room visits approximately one to two weeks following 12 and 18 month vaccination."[2] The researchers found that for every live vaccine given, there's one high-risk event to be expected for every 168 twelve-month-olds vaccinated, and one high-risk event for every 170 eighteen-month-old children vaccinated. Doctors expect to see twenty seizures for every 100,000 children vaccinated. Slowly it became evident to me that vaccinating our children is a shot in the dark, like playing the lottery using our children's lives.

If we're lucky, our child will not suffer from any short-term adverse reactions like seizures, disability, or death. But then again, what about long-term reactions? In an article by Edward L. Krawitt, Professor of Medicine at the University of Vermont's College of Medicine, I read: "Hepatitis is a general term that means inflammation of the liver. There are many forms and causes of hepatitis (such as viruses and certain drugs), including autoimmune hepatitis. In autoimmune hepatitis, the body's immune system attacks the cells of the liver, which causes the liver to become inflamed."[3]

The question is: Does a vaccine given to manipulate the immune system cause the cells to attack their own?

Yes. An article posted in the *Journal of Nature Medicine* reported that "aluminum in vaccines causes cell death."[4]

Another article states, "In the case of cell death from the vaccine adjuvant aluminum, the cell comes apart, releases DNA and other cell bits, and cannot be cleaned up easily. Cells neither break down in a controlled manner, nor do they send the appropriate signals for cleanup. This kind of cell death is called necrosis, and it's what can result in gangrene. An autoimmune disorder is a result of damage caused by an immune system that's gone awry, attacking part of its own body."[5]

Had I known that vaccines could cause unpredictable damage in children and that adjuvants used in vaccines had the potential of causing the immune system to attack its own cells (as in type-1 diabetes and other autoimmune disorders), I would have never exposed my children to vaccines, and I am convinced that I would have spared my daughter the torture of a life-long autoimmune disorder.

I wonder why it was that as a parent, I hadn't been informed in greater detail that vaccines had the potential of causing incredible harm to my children. Why was it that pediatricians and pediatric nurses, the people to whom we had entrusted our children's health, didn't engage us in a dialogue, pointing out the potential adverse events in order for us to make a well-informed decision? Why was it that any drug commercial on TV informed me of most possible, even unlikely side effects, but only a few were mentioned as far as vaccines were concerned?

The following pages provide more information and resources to help you answer these questions, but more importantly, they may provide you with lifesaving information that you would never hear from your pediatrician, pediatric nurse, or general practitioner.

The Known and Unknown

In order to make a decision on whether to have our children immunized, we need to look at what we know about vaccines and what we don't know about vaccines.

What we *know:*

1. Vaccines damage children shortly after they have been injected with a vaccine. This is called a short-term adverse reaction. The US government maintains a database that keeps track of injures and deaths due to vaccines.

2. Studies in natural settings have shown that the flu vaccine is worthless. By natural setting I mean a place where the flu reoccurs every year (retirement homes, public locations, etc.). People who have been immunized for the flu are as likely to get the flu as people who aren't immunized. "BEFORE the CDC advocated vaccinating children under the age of five, the number of children dying from the flu was very low, and on the decline. Then, in 2003, just after children aged five and under started getting vaccinated, the number of flu deaths SKYROCK-ETED. The death toll was enormous compared to the previous year, when the flu vaccine was not administered en masse to that age group."[6]

3. Vaccines are never tested against real, saline-only placebos in safety studies. The "placebos" given to the control groups are aluminum shots, thimerosal shots, or other vaccines.[7]

4. Scientists don't know if a vaccine is safe, because they don't do the necessary studies, and the studies they do perform aren't done with proper controls. What parents really want to know is the difference in side effects between getting the vaccine and not getting the vaccine. Unfortunately, the vast majority of people believe that this is actually tested. However, it isn't. Safety studies of the final product should only compare it to a true, saline-only placebo.[8]

5. Most parents take their children for multiple shots to the pediatrician without having ever taken a look at vaccine-package inserts, and have no idea what is given to their children and how it will affect them short-term and long-term.

6. According to the US Food and Drug Administration, "safety assessments for vaccines have not included appropriate toxicity studies because vaccines have not been viewed as inherently toxic."[9] In other words, our government based their claim that vaccines are safe on faith alone. This is what you subject your children to when going for your immunization appointment.

What we *don't know:*

7. Whether vaccines actually work. That is, we do not know whether vaccines actually protect from diseases. There is insufficient evidence, supporting the effectiveness of vaccines. Most pediatricians believe in the myth of vaccines protecting children from disease, even though they will not be able to

show you one single, methodologically sound study proving their claim.

8. The full scope of vaccines' long-term effects on children. A May 2012 article on emedicine.medscape.com "Aluminum Toxicity" notes:

> Generally, the medical profession thinks of the dangers of vaccinations in terms of deaths or retardation due to adverse reactions to vaccinations. Many parents may think about autism concerns. Actually, the dangers of vaccinations are far more widespread and certain in two important ways. First, vaccinations interrupt normal immune development when given before immune system maturity. When given after, they serve to hyper-excite one facet of the immune system in its relation to four other stages of natural immune system response. Normally, the immune system goes from (a) you smelling a sick person to (b) contact with the mucus membranes to (c) the blood (the specific area targeted by vaccinations) to (d) byproducts of pathogen breakdown, which then requires activity in the body cells and the lymphatic system. When one part is over-excited, the others may not function adequately, and the one targeted is likely to react excessively and ineffectively, such as in the case of allergies and autoimmune disease.

> Second, vaccinations also deposit a foreign protein (or protein particle) and its attendant cocktail of chemicals (and possibly heavy metals) into

the body without natural processes (e.g. injury) to alert the body to repel any invaders. History has shown us sadly that these particles may end up deposited in the body somewhere—usually an already weak area.[10]

It seems what we know and what we don't know about vaccines are equally scary. In the following chapters, I will take a closer look at vaccine effectiveness and the malpractice of vaccine research with information supported by expert opinion and the personal stories of parents whose children have been seriously injured by vaccines.

Challenging Information

In a recent conversation, I complained to a colleague of mine that Americans aren't outspoken enough about the direction the nation has been taking recently.

He told me, "Markus, the vast majority of people aren't informed enough to voice their opinion." He referred to the evening news and a man-on-the-street segment. People leaving the polls were quizzed about the candidates and the issues and failed miserably. These people were not too uninformed to voice their opinions—they *had* opinions…sometimes strong ones, backed by deep emotion. And they *had* taken political action by voting. They *had* made a choice… The point of the video was to suggest that it was clearly an uninformed (or misinformed) choice. The implication seemed to be that the voters hadn't done any independent research and were simply going along with vague notions that they'd absorbed from those around them and from secondary media sources, rather than from actual news reports.

I think we encounter the same issue when talking about vaccines. Parents receive misleading information about vaccine safety and effectiveness, and based on this misinformation, they decide to have their children vaccinated. In medicine as in politics, it's impossible to make an informed decision without first taking the time to become informed. The difference is that, while a misinformed voter may elect a bad candidate, two or four years later, he can vote again and correct his mistake.

A misinformed parent who makes a bad choice about vaccinations may never get a second chance.

As I was impatiently sitting in the waiting room of my GI doctor not too long ago, I wondered why I was the last patient that day, and why the whole process couldn't be any slower (as a German-American, I love sarcasm). I was scheduled to run a 5k the next day, and as I had been training on treadmills for the past five months, the transition to the road would be tough, so I really wanted to get in another run that day. My wife had taken our children to the in-laws for a little vacation, so I was free to run in the afternoon, but this was not meant to be—it was four-thirty before I was finally called into the office.

I had read my medical records and the latest research on my condition in order to have a beneficial discussion. My GI doctor is about my age. I like him a lot, as I find him better trained and more informed than my previous doctor, who recently retired.

Three weeks earlier, he had performed an upper endoscopy, which had involved stretching my esophagus and taking a biopsy. So now, during my late-afternoon appointment, he told me he'd come up with a new diagnosis and treatment plan. Based on the research I had conducted, I found his diagnosis to be valid.

A few minutes into our conversation, he said: "You are well read. I believe you are not the average patient." He went on his computer and pulled up some scientific articles, which we read together. This was a database only accessible to doctors; I thought out loud: "I wish

I had access to this. I recently did a lot of research on vaccines."

He paused for a minute and started to say something. Then he said, "You're not…well, I'd better keep my mouth shut."

I finished the sentence for him in my mind: "…one of those anti-vaccine nut cases."

What I said aloud was, "I found that there is no double-blind controlled placebo study proving that vaccines are even effective."

His response: "Come on, we eradicated smallpox with vaccines."

My response: "There is only correlation to this claim, and you know very well that a correlation doesn't provide us with scientific evidence."

With that, he didn't respond any further. The only addition he had was at the end of our meeting: "You know the only thing I hate about vaccines?" he asked. "When I take my daughter to the pediatrician, and she's injected with four different vaccines and they charge me four administration fees."

I know now why I was late in this office that day. I was his last patient, and we sat and talked for a long time. The vaccine conversation would not have happened had I not been the last patient. I feel that his last comment was to regain control he had lost in his argument. If he couldn't respond to my claim that correlation doesn't provide us with scientific evidence, he regained control by telling me that he is in charge of having his own children injected with vaccines.

The vast majority of people take their children to the pediatrician for immunizations having been told that this is the right, safe, and necessary thing to do, yet most parents in America have never educated themselves and researched vaccines before subjecting their children to this medical intervention. When pediatricians are asked about vaccine safety and effectiveness, they will point to studies or websites sponsored by the pharmaceutical industry, the US government, or the American Academy of Pediatrics—all of which are uncritical and ill-informed about vaccine adjuvants, and tolerant of insufficient toxicity studies. We wouldn't turn to the tobacco industry for safety studies about smoking (though the tobacco industry sponsored plenty of them), so to become educated about vaccine safety and effectiveness, we need to turn to scientists and groups unaffiliated with the pharmaceutical industry.

It doesn't take a scientific mind to find the abundance of research suggesting that vaccines are not as safe as they are claimed to be by the vast majority of pediatricians, health-care providers, and local, state, and federal officials. I have found enough evidence to make me seriously doubt that vaccines protect people from any potential illness. There is not only enough evidence to suggest that vaccines are ineffective, but more importantly, there *is* enough evidence of vaccine-related injuries and deaths to suggest that we should halt immunization until further toxicity studies of vaccine adjuvants have been conducted.

First, though, we need to *know* if vaccines actually work and whether vaccines are safe. These studies need to be double-blind controlled studies, to ensure the accuracy of the results. So far there have been no such studies comparing the overall health of vaccinated children to that of unvaccinated children. Unfortunately, the American Academy of Pediatrics, the vast majority of pediatricians, and the government refuse to recognize the results of tests that have already been conducted and choose, instead, to simply *believe* in the safety of vaccines.

Vaccine Controversy

Medical professionals warn that diseases will return when vaccines vanish. This is more than questionable. Many adults in the United States have never been vaccinated at all or haven't received a booster shot. We are talking about millions and millions of adults who have never received a measles vaccine, or whose immunity wore off a long time ago. Despite many millions of unvaccinated adults in America, there hasn't been an outbreak of measles or any other disease among that age group. Despite millions of unvaccinated adults, diseases have not returned within this unvaccinated population. As I already said, the notion that diseases will return when we stop vaccinating is more than questionable and not supported by research.

I read an article about a ten-year-old boy who contracted meningitis. His legs and arms had to be amputated, as his tissue was eaten by bacteria. It is quite a fearful scenario to think that my children could endure the same fate.

According to the pro-vaccine factions in this country, had he been vaccinated, he would have only had a 15-percent chance of having contracted this disease. Stories like these push parents to submit without even questioning the possible safety issues of vaccines. Even a critical person like me gets touched emotionally, and the rational part of me has to struggle to keep control of my senses. Of course, we can't know whether this boy would have been protected by the vaccine, as there's no evidence that any vaccine protects from diseases.

Yes, children contract illnesses—that is a fact of life. But, there is a distinct difference between your child contracting an illness by chance and you, as a parent, causing your child to be severely handicapped by having him or her injected with vaccines. And, *most* illnesses strengthen the immune system and are no more than an inconvenience, whereas every vaccine injected into your child promises a half-life of four years for aluminum and cell damage.

> For example, there is the story of little Ben Zeller.[11] Ten days after his MMR vaccine, Ben began to suffer from seizures, and he is now permanently disabled. The family filed a lawsuit under the National Vaccine Injury Act of 1986 and proved that the vaccine had caused little Ben's permanent disability. Ultimately the court highlighted the fact that Ben had been progressing and was neurologically stable until he received the MMR vaccine. (Judge) Special Master Richard Abell noted that if regression had been occurring prior to the vaccination, there would be mention of it in the thorough documentation that was presented to the court. "The first note of regression noted in the medical records appears to be from December of 2004," read the entitlement ruling, "following the vaccination, the initial seizure ten days subsequent, and the bout of successive seizures

in early December. The medical progress notes from 17 December 2004 include a description of Benjamin's 'developmental regression and seizures.'" The court also found that neuro-degeneration was not taking place prior to the vaccination, as Wiznitzer postulated. "If not but for the administration of the vaccines, Ben would not have suffered brain damage and seizures". The Zeller family was awarded one of the largest settlements in vaccine court history.

Countless statements on the CDC (Center for Disease Control) and medical websites read that vaccines are the safest pharmaceutical products. But we don't know that, and for doctors and scientists to make that argument is nothing but absurd and misleading. They should know better. Studies conducted by the pharmaceutical industries are methodologically wrong and not designed to show whether vaccines are safe.

On the *VaccineXchange* I found a good example: "If a middle school student was to compare the effects of table salt on blood pressure and used sea salt or kosher salt as his control, we all can fairly safely predict that the student may find that table salt has no different effect on blood pressure than sea salt or kosher salt. Could this student then argue that table salt is safe"?[12] Can the pharmaceutical industry and your pediatrician argue that vaccines are safe when the vaccine your child is about to be injected with has only been tested against another vaccine rather than saline? No. Yet, this is exactly what happens.

Your pediatrician, scientists, and your government also claim that vaccines are safe based on post-vaccination reports. As a matter of fact, our government finds vaccines so incredibly safe that it established VAERS (Vaccine Adverse Event Reporting System) and VICP (Vaccine Injury Compensation Program). So far the United States government has paid out over $1 billion dollars to parents whose children have been injured by vaccines.

The American government also put a price tag on vaccine injuries. In the event that you or your child dies because of an adverse vaccination event, it is worth $250,000 to your government.[13] You can see the contradiction. Government officials, doctors, and other health professionals tell you that vaccines are safe, yet, they've established a program to reimburse for severe injuries or death caused by vaccines. And those programs only reimburse you for short-term adverse events. We will look at long-term adverse vaccine events later.

Let's again look at the definition of "safe". The Merriam Webster dictionary defines safe as "free from harm or risk." We already know vaccines are not free of harm or risk. How then can your pediatrician claim that vaccines are safe? How can government officials claim vaccines are safe, when at the same time, they establish a program to report and reimburse for adverse reactions and death?

How many reports does VAERS receive? About 30,000 reports are received by VAERS each year: 10–15% involve hospitalization, permanent disability, or are considered life-threatening; about 2% involve death.[14] At the same time it is estimated that only 1–10% of all doctors report a severe health problem that occurs after a drug or vaccine is given to a patient.[15]

> According to Miles Braun from the *Institute for Vaccine Safety*, "underreporting is an inherent problem of passive surveillance systems, including VAERS. The degree of underreporting varies according to the adverse event. For example, one study estimated that 68% of cases of vaccine-associated polio are reported to VAERS, but only 4% of MMR-associated thrombocytopenia are reported. This variability in underreporting can make it hazardous to assume that the relative frequencies of adverse events in VAERS reflect their relative rates of occurrence.[16]

We, therefore, have to estimate that there are more than the reported severe adverse events taking place in America every year. We also have to estimate that there are more than the reported vaccine induced illnesses occurring in America every year.

Again, keep in mind that we are only talking about adverse events taking place within seventy-two hours after vaccination—not long-term adverse events. The same government that claims vaccines are free of harm also provides a vaccine injury table. The Department of Health and Human Services states:

The Vaccine Injury Table makes it easier for some people to get compensation. The Table lists and explains injuries/conditions that are presumed to be caused by vaccines. It also lists time periods in which the first symptom of these injuries/conditions must occur after receiving the vaccine. If the first symptom of these injuries/conditions occurs within the listed time periods, it is presumed that the vaccine was the cause of the injury or condition unless another cause is found.[17]

Do Vaccines Work?

Let's use the flu vaccine as an example and look at sound scientific evidence. Who has this evidence? The Cochrane Collaboration! On their website, you can find out who they are:

> The Cochrane Collaboration, established in 1993, is an international network of more than 28,000 dedicated people from over 100 countries. We work together to help health-care providers, policy-makers, patients, their advocates and caregivers, make well-informed decisions about health care, based on the best-available research evidence, by preparing, updating, and promoting the accessibility of *Cochrane Reviews*—over 4,600 so far, published online in The Cochrane Library."[18]

Working for the Cochrane Collaboration, an epidemiologist named Dr. Tom Jefferson decided to take a close look at the scientific evidence behind influenza (seasonal flu) vaccines. The objectives of the study were to "identify, retrieve, and assess all studies evaluating the effects of vaccines against influenza in healthy adults."

The Search Criteria: "We searched the Cochrane Central Register of Controlled Trials (CENTRAL) (*The Cochrane Library,* 2010, issue 2), MEDLINE (January 1966 to June 2010), and EMBASE (1990 to June 2010)." Selection Criteria (for inclusion in the study): "Randomized controlled trials (RCTs) or quasi-RCTs comparing influenza vaccines with placebo or no intervention in naturally-occurring influenza in healthy individuals aged sixteen to sixty-five years. We also included comparative studies assessing serious and rare harms."

The total scope of Jefferson's study encompassed over 70,000 people. And just so you know, these results may strongly favor the vaccine industry. The author even went out of his way to warn that "fifteen out of thirty-six trials were funded by industry (four had no funding declaration)." In other words, close to half of the studies included in this analysis were funded by the vaccine industry itself.

The results of the study show: "The corresponding figures [of people showing influenza symptoms] for poor vaccine matching were 2% and 1% (RD 1, 95% CI 0% to 3%)." And by "poor vaccine matching," they mean that the strain of influenza viruses in the vaccine was a poor match for the strains circulating in the wild. This is the case in the real world, because the vaccine only incorporates last year's viral strains and cannot predict which strains will be circulating this year. In other words, you would have to vaccinate 100 people to reduce the number of people developing influenza symptoms by just one. "For ninety-nine percent of the people vaccinated, the vaccine makes no difference at all."[19]

We can simply conclude that, based on sound scientific research, the flu vaccine is worthless.

"Conventional medicine, they say, is really "Evidence-Based Medicine" (EBM). That is, everything promoted by conventional medicine is supposed to be based on "rigorous scientific scrutiny." It's all supposed to be statistically validated and proven beyond a shadow of a doubt that it works as advertised. And in the case of vaccines, they are advertised as providing some sort of absolute protection against diseases.

This implication is wildly inaccurate. In fact, it's just flat-out false. As you'll see below, it's false advertising wrapped around junk science.

There was also never an independent, randomized, double-blind, placebo-controlled study proving either the safety or effectiveness of the H1N1 swine flu vaccines that were heavily pushed last year (and are in fact in this year's flu-shot cocktail). No such study has ever been done. As a result, there is no rigorous scientific basis from which to sell such vaccines in the first place."[20] If there is no rigorous scientific basis to claim that vaccines work, why do government officials, pediatricians, and other health officials tell you they protect your child from harm? Why don't they push for more conclusive research? Here's the answer provided by Mike Adams:

> Because most doctors and the scientific community claims that it would be "unethical" to conduct a placebo-controlled study of vaccines because apparently vaccines work so well that to deny the placebo group the actual vaccine would be harmful to them. Everybody benefits from vaccines, they insist, so the mere act of conducting a scientifically-controlled test is unethical.[21]

The scientific community, however, has no problem withholding treatment from terminally ill people in other instances:

> The *New England Journal of Medicine* recently published two studies regarding post-heart-attack patient cooling, which seeks to minimize brain damage by physically lowering the temperature of the brain of the heart attack patient until they can reach the acute care technicians at a nearby hospital. In two studies, researchers who already knew that "cooling" would save lives nevertheless subjected 350 heart attack patient to a randomized study protocol that assigned comatose (but resuscitated) patients to either "cooling" temperatures or normal temperatures. In one study, while half the cooled patients recovered with normal brain function, only a quarter of those exposed to normal temperatures did. In other words, patient cooling saved their brains. And yet the importance of knowing whether or not this procedure really worked was apparently enough to justify withholding the treatment from over a hundred other patients, most of whom suffered permanent brain damage as a result.[22]

> Do you smell some quackery at work yet? Not wanting to do an independent, randomized, double-blind, placebo-controlled study is precisely the kind of pseudo-scientific gobbledygook you might hear from some mad Russian scientist

who claims to have "magic water," but you can't test the magic water because the mere presence of measurement instruments nullifies the magical properties of the water. Similarly, vaccine pushers often insist it's unethical to test whether their vaccines really work. You just have to "take it on faith" that vaccines are universally good for everybody.

Yep, I used the word, "faith." That is essentially what the so-called scientific community is invoking here with the vaccine issue: Just *believe* they work, everybody! Who needs scientific evidence when we've got *faith* in vaccines?"[23]

In summary, in a study using 70,000 people, it was found that the flu vaccine doesn't work, and yet your doctor tells you that he or she is opposed to Evidence Based Medicine and independent, randomized, double-blind, placebo-controlled studies proving either the safety or effectiveness of vaccines.

"We have an entire segment of the scientific community that has been suckered into vaccine propaganda," Jefferson concludes. "They've convinced themselves that seasonal flu shots really work, and that virtually everyone should be injected with such shots. And they believe this based on irrational faith, not on scientific thinking or rigorous statistical evidence."[24]

Let's take a look how foolish one can look when choosing irrational faith over scientific facts. I found a little story about two doctors believing in vaccine effectiveness.

Funny, Yet Serious

To all of you who have done research in this field, you will appreciate the irony of the following paragraph from an abstract in *The Journal of Infectious Diseases.* To all of you who have been conditioned to believe that vaccines actually protect your children from diseases and do no harm, hopefully you will appreciate the seriousness of the issue at hand.

The abstract reads,

> In 2009, measles outbreaks in Pennsylvania and Virginia resulted in the exposure and apparent infection of 2 physicians, both of whom had a documented history of vaccination with >2 doses of measles-mumps-rubella vaccine… both of the physicians continued to see patients, because neither considered that they could have measles.[25]

It is a funny but serious reality that the two physicians mentioned in the article didn't even *consider* the fact that they might have measles. The behavior of those two physicians is symptomatic for the vast majority of physicians in this country, who have been trained by pharmaceuticals-sponsored and-written textbooks and indoctrinated by flawed and scientifically unsound studies. Even when they had contracted the disease against which they had been vaccinated, they were unable to see the symptoms, even though they had been trained to detect them. This story practically defines the word *indoctrination.*

I can almost hear those measle-bearing doctors talking to concerned parents, reassuring them that vaccines work, and that they will protect their babies from harmful diseases like measles. I can see them storming madly out the room when confronted by parents expressing doubts that vaccines actually work, all the while mumbling that vaccines have protected millions of people from disease. But vaccines did not protect these two doctors. Did they protect anyone in the past? Let's take a look.

Did Diseases Decline Because of Vaccines?

Though there are no double-blind studies, or any long-term studies showing that vaccines confer immunity, doctors and health-care providers always put forth the argument that because of vaccines, previously deadly diseases have vanished or have been eradicated. This isn't really true, as the following graphs show. You can see that diseases had begun to decline prior to the introduction of the vaccines that "eradicated" them. As vaccines were introduced, the illnesses continued to decline, but concluding that the decline occurred because of vaccines is a pretty far stretch, as the decline clearly began before the vaccine was introduced.

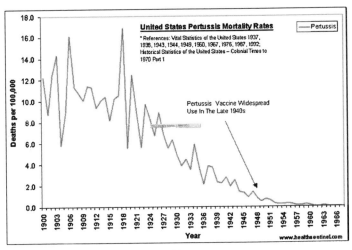

26

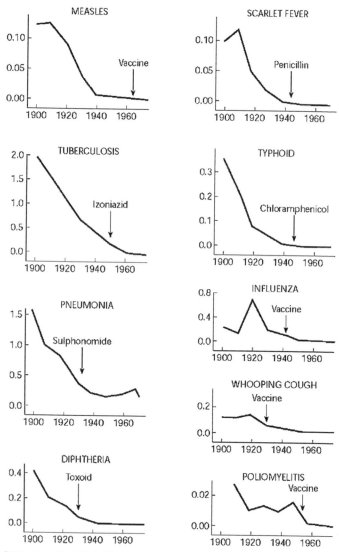

Figure 1.1 The fall in the standardized death rate (per 1000 population) for nine common infectious diseases in relation to specific medical measures in the USA, 1900–1973.
Source: McKinlay and McKinlay (1981).

27

43

Having questioned the effectiveness of vaccines, seriously doubting that they protect any children from harm, I now turn to the more important aspect of vaccines safety. It is one thing to have your child injected with a worthless substance; however, it is worse if your child gets hurt in the process.

Are Vaccines Safe?

Somewhere in America today, parents will take their most-precious possession to the pediatrician, thinking they are doing the right thing, completely unaware of any possible life-threatening side effects after immunization.

According to the Centers for Disease Control and Prevention (CDC) and the Food and Drug Administration (FDA), approximately 30,000 VAERS reports are filed annually, with 10-15% classified as serious, resulting in permanent disability, hospitalization, life-threatening illnesses or death.[28] And those are only the reported cases of vaccine induced deaths, disability, illness and hospitalization.

At www.rense.com, a mother states the following:

> Vaccines kill at a much higher rate than we are led to believe. We play vaccine roulette with our children's lives and we never know which child will fall victim next. If the odds are 1 in 500,000 for death, 1 in 100,000 for permanent brain injury, 1 in 1,700 for seizures and convulsions or 1 in 100 for adverse reaction, are you willing to take that chance? Are any odds acceptable enough to convince you to gamble with your child's life? I can assure you that death from vaccination is neither quick nor painless. I helplessly watched my daughter suffer an excruciatingly slow death as she screamed and arched her back in pain, while the vaccine did as it was intended to do and assaulted her immature immune system.

The poisons used as preservatives seeped through her tiny body, overwhelming her vital organs one by one until they collapsed. It is an image that will haunt me forever, and I hope no other parent ever has to witness it.[29]

Most children survive the first seventy-two hours after vaccination without obvious harm. But you are basically playing the lottery with your child's health and well-being, as there are tens of thousands documented short-term side effects ranging from seizures to deaths. Someone will get hurt.

There are no long-term studies within the medical community comparing unvaccinated children to vaccinated children. I find this absolutely irresponsible, as this provides us with no idea how vaccines affect our children in the long-run. A correlation study should be possible, as there are "3 in 1,000 children in America alone who never received a vaccine."[30] With roughly 41 million children aged 0–18 in America that would make the population of unvaccinated children about 120,000. That is a population large enough to obtain statistically sound results and rule out other factors that might skew or falsely impact the results.

At this point, I think it is also important to know that the US government handed the pharmaceutical industry a "blank check." When you see the next drug commercial on television or listen to it on the radio, simply pay attention to the side effects mentioned. Then wait for side effects to be mentioned when you hear the next announcement to immunize you children or yourself.

But don't hold your breath. Thanks to our government, pharmaceutical companies *cannot* be sued for adverse reactions due to vaccinations. They are exempt from lawsuits. If your child is hurt by a vaccine, the manufacturer of that vaccine bears no responsibility. You may draw your own conclusions and sue the government instead.

I found a study conducted in Germany by the famous Robert-Koch Institute (The German Health Interview and Examination Survey for Children and Adolescents).[31] The study was conducted between 2003 and 2006. There were 17,641 participants who finished the study. Of those 17,641 participants, 134 were completely unvaccinated. Even though this study was not meant to compare the health of vaccinated versus unvaccinated children, it provided an excellent opportunity to do so, as the parents indicated whether their children were or were not vaccinated, along with a detailed health status of their children. I then looked for someone who took on the work of comparing vaccination status to health. I came across the website of a German mathematician and computer scientist who analyzed the report. After publication of her findings in June 2009, she received a phone call from the Robert-Koch Institute (similar to the US Center for Disease Control) and was unethically attacked for apparently wrongly interpreting the numbers.[32]

The Robert-Koch Institute vowed to work on a rebuttal and publish it in the German medical journal by 2010. We are now in 2012, and still anxiously await the rebuttal. In the meantime, here are some results of the study:

Allergies in Vaccinated versus Unvaccinated Children

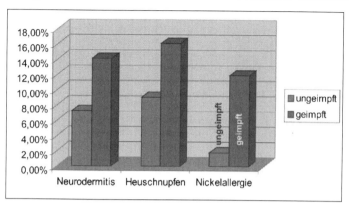

ungeimpft = unvaccinated

geimpft = vaccinated

Neurodermitis = eczema

Heuschnupfen = hay fever

Nickelallergie = nickel allergy

Illness in Vaccinated versus Unvaccinated Children

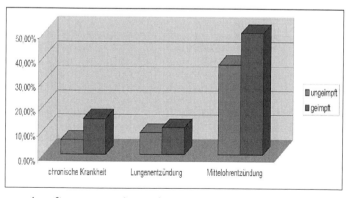

ungeimpft = unvaccinated

geimpft = vaccinated

chronische Krankheit = chronic disease

Lungenentzündung = pneumonia

Mittelohrentzündung = ear infections

Average Number of Infections the Year after Vaccination

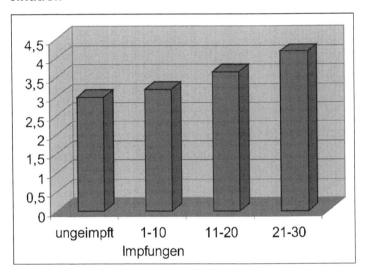

ungeimpft = unvaccinated

Impfungen = Vaccines

More vaccines = more infections

Source: http://www.gesundheitlicheaufklaerung.de/impfen-macht-krank

The graphs show clearly that vaccinated children tended to have more infections, allergies, and chronic illnesses. I have observed the very same phenomenon in our children. In the months after vaccines have been given,

our children had ear infections, upper respiratory infections, and colds. The more time passes between vaccines given, the less infections occur. Yet, our daughter
Johanna is now "stuck" with an autoimmune disorder
that started after her last set of vaccines.

Various Vaccines and the Damage they Cause

The National Library of Medicine contains the findings from some very specific research studies that reveal the dangers vaccines can pose to our children's health.

The HPV Vaccine

In "Human papillomavirus (HPV) vaccine policy and evidence-based medicine: Are they at odds?" Shaw Tomljenovic writes,

> All drugs are associated with some risks of adverse reactions. Because vaccines represent a special category of drugs, generally given to healthy individuals, uncertain benefits mean that only a small level of risk for adverse reactions is acceptable. Furthermore, medical ethics demand that vaccination should be carried out with the participant's full and informed consent. This necessitates an objective disclosure of the known or foreseeable vaccination benefits and risks. The way in which HPV vaccines are often promoted to women indicates that such disclosure isn't always given from the basis of the best-available knowledge. For example, while the world's leading medical authorities state that HPV vaccines are an important cervical cancer prevention tool, clinical trials show no evidence that HPV vaccination can protect against cervical cancer. Similarly, contrary to claims that cervical

cancer is the second-most common cancer in women worldwide, existing data show that this only applies to developing countries. In the Western world, cervical cancer is a rare disease with mortality rates that are several times lower than the rate of reported serious adverse reactions (including deaths) from HPV vaccination. Future vaccination policies should adhere more rigorously to evidence-based medicine and ethical guidelines for informed consent.[33]

Vaccines and Autism

In "Do Aluminum Vaccine Adjuvants Contribute to the Rising Prevalence of Autism?" the researchers found that "data indicates that the correlation between Al in vaccines and ASD may be causal."[34] The abstract for the study summarizes its findings thusly:

Autism spectrum disorders (ASD) are serious multisystem developmental disorders and an urgent global public health concern. Dysfunctional immunity and impaired brain function are core deficits in ASD. Aluminum (Al), the most commonly used vaccine adjuvant, is a demonstrated neurotoxin and a strong immune stimulator. Hence, adjuvant Al has the potential to induce neuroimmune disorders. When assessing adjuvant toxicity in children, two key points ought to be considered: (i) children should not be viewed as "small adults," as their unique physiology makes them much more vulnerable to toxic insults; and (ii) if exposure to Al from only a few vaccines can lead to cognitive impairment and autoimmunity in adults, is it unreasonable to question whether the current pediatric schedules, often containing eighteen Al adjuvanted vaccines, are safe for children? By applying Hill's criteria for establishing causality between exposure and outcome, we investigated whether exposure to Al from vaccines could be contributing to the rise in ASD prevalence in the Western world. Our results show that: (i) children from countries with the highest ASD prevalence appear to have the highest exposure to Al from vaccines; (ii) the increase in exposure to Al adjuvants significantly correlates with the increase in ASD prevalence in the United States observed over the last two decades (Pearson r=0.92, p<0.0001); and (iii) a significant correlation exists between the amounts of Al administered to preschool children and the current prevalence of ASD in seven Western countries, particularly at 3–4 months of age (Pearson r=0.89-0.94, p=0.0018-0.0248). The application of the Hill's criteria to these data indicates that the correlation between Al in vaccines and ASD may be causal. Because children represent a fraction of the population most at risk for complications following exposure to Al, a more-rigorous evaluation of Al adjuvant safety seems warranted.[36]

Hepatitis B Vaccine

In "A Case-Control Study of Serious Autoimmune-Adverse Events Following Hepatitis B Immunization," we find that "Adults receiving HBV had significantly increased odds ratios (OR) for multiple sclerosis (OR = 5.2, $p < 0.0003$, 95% Confidence Interval [CI] = 1.9–20), optic neuritis (OR = 14, $p < 0.0002$, 95% CI = 2.3 - 560), vasculitis (OR = 2.6, $p < 0.04$, 95% CI = 1.03 - 8.7), arthritis (OR = 2.01, $p < 0.0003$, 95% CI = 1.3–3.1), alopecia (OR = 7.2, $p < 0.0001$, 95% CI = 3.2–20), lupus erythematosus (OR = 9.1, $p < 0.0001$, 95% CI = 2.3 - 76), rheumatoid arthritis (OR = 18, $p < 0.0001$, 95% CI = 3.1–740), and thrombocytopenia (OR = 2.3, $p < 0.04$, 95% CI = 1.02–6.2)",[36] clearly showing the statistical evidence of the risk this particular vaccine causes.

Vaccines and Autoimmune Syndrome

Researchers have proposed a new syndrome potentially caused by vaccines, or more specifically, by vaccine adjuvants or preservatives. With regards to vaccines causing autoimmune diseases and this newly proposed syndrome, the researchers write:

> There has been considerable interest in the role of environmental factors and the induction of autoimmunity and the ways by which they facilitate loss of tolerance. Clearly both genetic and environmental factors are incriminated, as evidenced by the lack of concordance in identical twins and the relatively recent identification of the shared epitope in rheumatoid arthritis. In this issue a new syndrome called "Asia'-autoimmune/auto-inflammatory syndrome induced by adjuvants has been proposed. It is an intriguing issue and one that is likely to be provocative and

lead to further biologic and molecular investigations.[37]

What I find particularly interesting is that even some researchers whom I perceive as being pro-vaccination admit the potential of vaccines causing autoimmune diseases. For instance, after claiming, "Universal vaccination remains the most effective way of preventing the spread of many infectious diseases," Z. Karali admits, "Although most adverse effects attributed to vaccines are mild, rare reactions such as autoimmunity do occur."[38]

Scientifically Wrong Vaccine Safety Studies

Any trained scientist or statistician understands that you want to use a *null hypothesis* to disprove a possible causal relationship between two correlated events. The null hypothesis in this case would be: There is no causal connection between vaccinations and their alleged adverse short-term and long-term side effects.

If we were going to test this hypothesis, I would randomly sample research subjects (a large sample size of perhaps 100,000 would help exclude other factors) and divide the subjects into two groups. One group will get the vaccine, and the other group would receive a saline shot. Both groups would then be monitored for at least four weeks to observe whether short-term side effects were more prevalent in the vaccinated group than in the placebo group.

To determine whether or not there is a causal link between vaccinations and long-term medical complications would be a little more difficult. Nonetheless, if one group of subjects has received a placebo and the other has received the vaccine, it would be possible to mail a questionnaire to randomly selected parents who have chosen to immunize their children and to an equal-sized group of those who haven't. A phone interview could also take place. This would be a good starting point to see whether there are differences in the long-term health and development of vaccinated children versus that of non-vaccinated children. If no significant differences are found between the two groups in either the short term or long term, then the pro-vaccine factions can rejoice, because they've disproven the anti-vaccinators' claims and proved that the vaccine in question does not cause short-term or long-term complications.

If researchers wanted to know the truth about vaccines' effects, it would be easy enough to discover. Let's take a look at what methodology the pharmaceutical industries use to obtain the results they desire. Here it is, as explained in the package inserts for the hepatitis B vaccine by GlaxoSmithKline:

> Ten double-blind studies involving 2,252 subjects showed no significant difference in the frequency or severity of adverse experiences between ENGERIX-B and plasma-derived vaccines.

> In thirty-six clinical studies, a total of 13,495 doses of ENGERIX-B were administered to 5,071 healthy adults and children who were initially seronegative for hepatitis B markers and healthy neonates. All subjects were monitored for four days post-administration.

What the pharmaceutical company *should* have done is inject one group with the vaccine and the other group with a non-vaccine placebo (i.e., saline). What the pharmaceutical company did, instead, was inject one group with the hepatitis B vaccine, and the other group with *a different vaccine*. Then they monitored both groups and found that the recipients of their vaccine had "no significant difference in the frequency or severity of adverse experiences" as compared to the recipients of other vaccines. Which tells us nothing, really. Imagine McDonald's touting their Big Macs as being "no more lethal than the Whopper."

This is exactly what the pharmaceutical company has done here—they've avoided the real question about adverse reactions to vaccinations by announcing that their vaccine causes no more adverse reactions than other vaccines. But make no mistake about it, adverse reactions occurred in both groups.

Let's take a close look at the package inserts of various drug companies and the vaccines they manufacture. More importantly, let's look at how the pharmaceutical companies manipulate safety results.

Sanofi Pasteur and the HIB Vaccine

> In a randomized, double-blind US clinical trial, ActHIB vaccine was given concomitantly with DTP to more than 5,000 infants, and hepatitis B vaccine was given with DTP to a similar number. In this large study, deaths due to sudden infant death syndrome (SIDS) and other causes were observed, but were not different in the two groups. In the first forty-eight hours following immunization, two definite and three possible seizures were observed after ActHIB vaccine and DTP in comparison with none after hepatitis B vaccine and DTP.[39]

In order for us to know how safe the HIB vaccine is, the vaccine should have been compared to a placebo.

Only then would we know how safe the vaccine truly is. But in order to muddy the results, not only did they not compare the HIB vaccine to a placebo, but they combined the HIB vaccine with another vaccine, and then tested it against two *other* combined vaccines. Imagine a drug company testing the safety of infant Tylenol by mixing it with another drug and then comparing it to a mixture of two other drugs. How would we ever be able to tell whether Tylenol is safe to give to our children?

Merck and Hepatitis B Vaccine

> In the pivotal, randomized, multicenter study, 882 infants were assigned in a 3:1 ratio to receive either COMVAX or PedvaxHIB plus RECOMBIVAX HB at separate injection sites at 2, 4, and 12–15 months of age. Children may have also received routine pediatric immunizations. The children were monitored daily for five days after each injection for injection-site and systemic adverse experiences. During this time, adverse experiences in infants who received COMVAX were generally similar in type and frequency to those observed in infants who received PedvaxHIB plus RECOMBIVAX HB.[40]

In this study, Merck figured it would be best to compare its hepatitis B vaccine to a mixture of two other vaccines. Why would they do this? Because if a single vaccine is compared to a mixture of vaccines, the likelihood of adverse reactions in the "mixture of vaccine group" is likely to be higher, therefore making the hepatitis B vaccine look relatively safe. This is manipulation at its best.

Sanofi Pasteur and the Polio Vaccine

In earlier studies with the vaccine grown in primary monkey kidney cells, transient local reactions at the site of injection were observed. Erythema, induration and pain occurred in 3.2%, 1% and 13%, respectively, of vaccinees within 48 hours post-vaccination. Temperatures of ≥39°C (≥102°F) were reported in 38% of vaccinees. Other symptoms included irritability, sleepiness, fussiness, and crying. Because IPV was given in a different site but concurrently with diphtheria and tetanus toxoids and pertussis vaccine adsorbed (DTP), these systemic reactions could not be attributed to a specific vaccine. However, these systemic reactions were comparable in frequency and severity to that reported for DTP given alone without IPV. Although no causal relationship has been established, deaths have occurred in temporal association after vaccination

of infants with IPV.[41]

It is interesting to know that the vaccine grows in monkey kidney cells. I wonder what impact this has on our children. In this study, the pharmaceutical company tells us that the experienced side effects can't be attributed to the polio vaccines, as it was tested by mixing the polio vaccine and then comparing it to the mixture of two other vaccines. This is simply beyond words.

All the package inserts can be accessed by going to: http://www.vaccinesafety.edu/package_inserts.htm.

In order to show how ridiculously vaccine safety studies are designed, here is a comparison: I want to find out whether eating huge quantities of Hershey kisses can lead to a bellyache. What I should do is get two groups of large sizes together and give one group large amounts of Hershey kisses and the other group a placebo. If there are significantly more bellyaches in the Hershey kiss group, I can confidently say that it isn't safe to eat large quantities of Hershey kisses. Instead, I randomly sample two large groups and give one group large quantities of Hershey kisses and the other group large quantities of gummy bears or, perhaps, as some study designs by the pharmaceutical industry suggest, the placebo group receives large quantities of gummy bears and ice cream at the same time. Now I have belly aches in both groups (as we all know eating too much chocolate or gummy bears isn't good), however, because I have an equal amount of reactions in both groups, I argue that it is therefore safe to eat large amounts of Hershey kisses, as there are not significantly more bellyaches in the Hershey kiss group.

This is how the pharmaceutical industry conducts their double-blind pseudo studies to prove that vaccines are safe.

In the following chapters I will take you behind the scene. I will introduce you to vaccine scientists and developers and vaccine promoters. I will ask the question how credible the pro-vaccine community is compared to those who think of vaccines critically, ending with doctors who left the vaccination bandwagon and their reasons for doing so.

Dr. Maurice Hilleman versus Your Pediatrician—A Comparison

It doesn't happen very often that a vaccine expert speaks freely about the safety of vaccines. One of the leading vaccine experts was Dr. Maurice Hilleman.

Who was Dr. Hilleman exactly? Author Cynthia Janak provides a brief biography:

> Dr. Hilleman was, and is, the leading vaccine pioneer in the history of vaccines. He developed more than three dozen vaccines—more than any other scientist in history—and was the developer of Merck's vaccine program.
>
> He was a member of the US National Academy of Science, the Institute of Medicine, the American Academy of Arts and Sciences, and the American Philosophical Society, and received a special lifetime achievement award from the World Health Organization.
>
> When he was chief of the Department of Respiratory Diseases with what's now the Walter Reed Army Institute of Research, he discovered the genetic changes that occur when the influenza virus mutates, known as *shift and drift*. He was also one of the early vaccine pioneers to warn about the possibility that simian viruses might contaminate vaccines.[42]

So, on one hand, we have your average pediatrician ensuring you that vaccines are safe. This assurance is based on "theoretical knowledge" your pediatrician has acquired. On the other hand, we have the leading vaccine pioneer who has been in the lab experimenting and working in the field of vaccine research and development. Based on his work, Dr. Maurice Hilleman warned that vaccines are contaminated with lethal viruses.

> A measles vaccine was found to contain low levels of the retrovirus avian leukosis (AVL) virus— a virus known to cause cancer in chickens. This despite the fact that vaccine manufacturers have been required to use eggs from leukosis-free stocks for over forty years. Rotateq, Merck's rotavirus vaccine, was found to contain a virus similar to simian (monkey) retrovirus—the SV40 virus previously linked to human cancer.[43]

> In 2002, the journal *Lancet* published compelling evidence that a contaminated polio vaccine was responsible for up to half of the 55,000 non-Hodgkin's lymphoma cases that were occurring each year. The puzzle began in 1994, when Dr. Michele Carbone, a Loyola University researcher, found the virus SV40, which had never before been detected in humans, in half of the human lung tumors he was studying. Since then, sixty different lab studies have confirmed the results, and SV40 has been found in a variety of human cancers, including lung-, brain-, bone-, and lymphatic cancer. At first, no one could fathom how

the virus had been transmitted into the human population. But in the censored interview with Dr. Maurice Hilleman above, Hilleman admits Merck's responsibility in unleashing this virus via their polio vaccine, as well as the likelihood that there was an importing and of spreading the AIDS virus in the same manner.[44]

Dr. Hilleman also warned that vaccines can cause the very disease they are supposed to prevent. This is the case with the polio vaccine. There are no cases of wild polio (naturally caused polio) left in the United States. Instead we now see elevated numbers of vaccine-induced polio.

Naturalnews.com reports the following on this issue:

> One of the most prominent vaccine scientists in the history of the vaccine industry—a Merck scientist—made a recording where he openly admits that vaccines given to Americans were contaminated with leukemia and cancer viruses. In response, his colleagues (who are also recorded) break out into laughter and seem to think it's hilarious. They then suggest that because these vaccines are first tested in Russia, they will help the US win the Olympics because the Russian athletes will all be "loaded down with tumors."
>
> (Thus, *knew* these vaccines caused cancer in humans).
>
> This isn't some conspiracy theory—these are the words of a top Merck scientist who probably

had no idea that his recording would be widely reviewed across the Internet (which didn't even exist when he made this recording). He probably thought this would remain a secret forever. When asked why this didn't get out to the press, he replied, "Obviously you don't go out; this is a scientific affair within the scientific community." In other words, vaccine scientists cover for vaccine scientists. They keep all their dirty secrets within their own circle of silence and don't reveal the truth about the contamination of their vaccines.[45]

Dr. Maurice Hilleman provides us with the reality of vaccine safety issues, whereas your average pediatrician gives you the sugar-coated version. Dr. Hilleman's insights explain perfectly the rise in autoimmune disorders and childhood cancers we are experiencing since the introduction of mass vaccination. According to Dr. Hilleman's revelations, the scientific vaccine community seems to be aware of the risks vaccines pose. However, the concern of this scientific community is not particularly with your child, but with the continuation of a vaccination program that bears immense known and unknown risks. But the risks Dr. Maurice Hilleman referred to are all too visible in most vaccine inserts. You're left with a little yellow slip informing you of minor side effects. As a parent, it is up to you to choose in whom you place your trust when it comes to the safety of your child. Yes, your unvaccinated child may contract a disease naturally, but injecting a cancer virus into your child is a whole different story.

Strong Opposition – Why Vaccines are Promoted

Those of us who oppose the unreliable science advocating vaccine safety and effectiveness are few and far between. We are opposed by strong pro-vaccine fractions that have the money to get their message out to the public more effectively than we can. People like me are independent, and we have no conflicts of interest—only the desire to share what we have learned through diligent research.

This, however, cannot be said about most of the "independent experts" siding with the government and pharmaceutical companies advocating and promoting vaccines.

One of those prominent experts, Dr. Paul A. Offit, a paid employee of the Children's Hospital of Philadelphia, has a tremendous interest in vaccinating every child in America. In fact, he is so concerned that he's written books to try to convince us that vaccines are good for our children: *Vaccinated: One Man's Quest to Defeat the World's Deadliest Diseases; Vaccines and Your Child: Separating Fact from Fiction;* and *Deadly Choices: How the Anti-Vaccine Movement Threatens Us All.*

Even the titles of these books give us a fairly good idea about his objectives. This prominent researcher and pediatrician also patented a Rotavirus vaccine. Unfortunately, Offit's vaccine was withdrawn after 202 infant deaths were associated with it (as of September 2011).[46]

By then, however, our prominent expert had earned millions of dollars from his vaccine. Why didn't the Federal Drug Administration (FDA) catch on to the danger of this vaccine? The FDA didn't catch on because in the actual FDA study submitted by Merck, the company compared the vaccine to an undisclosed biological agent, rather than saline.[47] We have learned in previous chapters how those studies are designed and why they don't reveal all the dangers vaccines pose.

The other possibility is that our government is willing to accept deaths by vaccine as long as the majority of children don't die. The government as well as the pharmaceutical industry knew that hundreds of children would die from this Rotavirus vaccine. How do we know this? The clinical studies Merck conducted and submitted to the government agency for approval clearly state:

> 71,725 infants were evaluated in three placebo-controlled clinical trials including 36,165 infants in the group that received RotaTeq and 35,560 infants in the group that received placebo... Across the clinical studies, 52 deaths were reported. There were 25 deaths in the RotaTeq recipients compared to 27 deaths in the placebo recipients.["][48]

What information do we get from this study? We learn that

> (1) Merck used placebos that are more dangerous than the vaccine itself (25 deaths in vaccine group versus 27 deaths in placebo group), and

(2) the pharmaceutical company producing this vaccine and the FDA knew that many children would die from this vaccine. (When 36,165 children received this vaccine, 25 died. Statistically, this implied that if 361,650 children received this vaccine, it would kill 250 children.)

I haven't even mentioned other serious complications children experienced from this vaccine. Here's the takeaway: While most children who received RotaTeq didn't die or experience serious short-term complications, this was simply because they were lucky—not because their parents had made an informed decision.

Let's turn our attention again to one of America's biggest vaccine promoters: our expert, Paul Offit. He isn't only a pediatrician advising other pediatricians, he was also investigated by Congress for voting himself rich as a member of the US Advisory Committee on Immunization Practices (ACIP). Our expert voted for his own patented vaccine Rotavirus to be introduced into the US children's vaccine schedule when he was supposed to be objectively looking out for the health and safety of US children. He has made millions of dollars from the patent for the vaccine which he held in partnership with vaccine-maker Merck before the vaccine was withdrawn because more children died of the vaccine than the disease.

The congressional report shows that our expert:

- had already been awarded the patent on the rotavirus vaccine, which he shares in development with Merck

- received a $350,000 grant from Merck for rotavirus-vaccine development

- acts as a consultant to Merck

- voted yes three out of four times pertaining to the ACIP's rotavirus statement, including voting for the inclusion of the Rotavirus vaccine in the VFC program

- abstained from voting on the ACIP's rescission of its recommendation of the Wyeth rotavirus vaccine for routine use when serious adverse reactions were being reported. He stated at the meeting, "I'm not conflicted with Wyeth, but because I consult with Merck on the development of rotavirus vaccine, I would still prefer to abstain because it creates a perception of conflict.☐[49]

The next time your pediatrician informs you about the safety and effectiveness of vaccines, please remember this background information. Keep in mind that vaccines are put on the market knowing children will die from them and also keep in mind that those who educate pediatricians and the greater public about vaccines have and will continue to become very wealthy from their sale. Asking your pediatrician about the safety of vaccines is like asking a liquor store owner about the safety of the Marlboros he sells. Whatever he knows about Marlboros, he has probably learned from the Marlboro sales representative, who was trying to get him to buy her company's cigarettes. And where did the sale representative get her information? From the cigarette company itself.

Look for independent and unbiased sources. *Every* child has the right to be safe and protected by his or her parents. However, only informed parents can protect their children. As I have just questioned the credibility of a prominent vaccine researcher we will look at the credibility I bring to the table, especially in comparison to health officials promoting vaccines. But before I do that I am concluding with a book review. Dr. Russel L. Blaylock, a board-certified neurosurgeon, educator, and lecturer, comments on one of the above-mentioned titles, by Paul Offit:

> This book is nothing but a prolonged advertisement for the vaccine manufacturers from a physician who has profited handsomely from his own personally developed vaccine. There are a number of gross errors in the book and a slanderous attack on all the people who have formed groups to educate the public about vaccine dangers and the overstated efficacy of these vaccines. The so-called "anti-vaccine" people actually contain many who do not oppose vaccines, if they are safe and effective and the indications are justified. These individuals are mostly very intelligent, dedicated people who do extensive research and have the aid of some of the most well-respected researchers in the world.
>
> Many have had their children destroyed by these vaccines. Offit admits that he knows nothing about the neurological sciences, yet he boldly states that there is no mechanism to explain how

vaccines could harm the brain. There are a number of well-researched studies that clearly outline such a mechanism, explaining in accepted scientific terms why exposing small children and newborns to extremely high doses of known neurotoxins in repeated doses can result in abnormal brain development and prolonged neurological pathological change. The fact that children are given numerous vaccines during a single office visit and that this schedule is repeated every two months for the first two years of life defies what we know concerning excessive immune stimulation on the rapidly developing brain. Defenders of this dangerous vaccine policy, such as our expert, cannot justify what they are proposing and doing. The science is heavily on the side of those of us who insist on vaccine safety, efficacy, and informed consent. This book is filled with poor science, verbal attacks on decent people, and propaganda for the vaccine manufacturers.[50]

Credibility Issues

Is *this* book based on credible information? Am I, the author, credible? How credible is your pediatrician, the Center for Disease Control, the Federal Drug Administration? When pediatricians and scientists are confronted by inquisitive parents, they counter by either saying that parents (1) should only look at credible sources and not at "other peoples' comments," or argue that parents (2) aren't medical professionals and have no medical or scientific training to look into vaccine safety or effectiveness. They may say that only medical doctors are qualified to read and interpret clinical studies.

Not true. A study's sample size, design, and results are all aspects that are fairly simple to understand and interpret. In combination with available information from credible agencies and studies the credibility factor increases. Not only have I looked at an abundance of studies done by credible institutions and scientists, I have also listened and read statements from qualified medical professionals and scientists confirming my interpretation of the studies I have read. The problem of credibility clearly lies with your pediatrician telling you that studies have clearly shown that since the introduction of vaccines diseases declined, that vaccines are safe beyond doubt, and that vaccines work beyond any doubt. All of these claims have no well designed study supporting your pediatricians' claim.

Your pediatrician may also say that it would be "unethical" to withhold vaccines from children in a study comparing vaccinated to unvaccinated children. Here are the problems with that line of argument:

9. There are plenty of ongoing clinical studies where possibly lifesaving treatments are being withheld from people in order to test the safety and effectiveness of the treatments.

10. Withholding a vaccine for a few days is not unethical if doing so is needed in order to study its short-term side effects. If anything, it's unethical to license a vaccine that has killed several babies during clinical trials.

Here is an example regarding the effectiveness of vaccines. This is from a German website that uses information from the Robert-Koch Institute, the equivalent of the American CDC (Centers for Disease Control):

> Conclusively a study of vaccinated versus an unvaccinated population should exist in order to determine if vaccines are effective (meaning they actually work). This study should take place on a large scale over a long period of time and should be designed as double-blind and placebo controlled. Such studies, however, don't exist. Instead, scientists and doctors measure antibodies, or more specifically, the quantity of antibodies in the bloodstream. Your pediatrician will tell you that the presence and quantity of such antibodies prove the effectiveness of the vaccine.[51]

This is as far as your pediatrician will go, or the vaccine expert will argue, as they leave out an important bit of information: A missing titer (concentration of antibodies) doesn't mean that there's no immunity present in the organism. That is because of cellular immunity, which is independent of antibodies and constitutes a different part of the immune system. It is therefore possible to have immunity without measurable antibody titer.

Nevertheless, pediatricians and vaccine experts consistently refer to a high number of antibodies as a guarantee of immunity. Unfortunately there is no clinical study showing that a high number of antibodies guarantee immunity. Therefore, your pediatrician's rationale:

vaccines = creation of antibodies = immunity

is based on faith rather than clinical studies. As a parent, I am not willing to expose my children to a medical intervention based on good faith.

What about doctors? Aren't they violating the Hippocratic Oath by basing medical decisions on good faith?

Pediatricians, Vaccines, and the Hippocratic Oath

Does administering vaccines violate the Hippocratic Oath that doctors and most medical professionals have to take? A part of the oath reads:

- I will remember that there is art to medicine as well as science, and that warmth, sympathy, and understanding may outweigh the surgeon's knife or the chemist's drug.[52]

As a parent, I am an avid reader of articles submitted to me via email by www.babycenter.com. One of those articles, titled "7 signs of a bad doctor," sparked my interest. The article states:

> Consider changing doctors if yours—or your child's—doesn't seem to keep up with the latest medical literature or be aware of medical breakthroughs or other health information. Part of the job is to educate patients about their health. That means explaining the results of medical tests, *keeping patients informed about drugs prescribed,* and providing nutrition and other health advice.[53]

The pediatricians we have seen with our children have never informed us of *all* possible side effects of vaccines. Yes, we received a little yellow paper mentioning a few possible side effects, but by no means did they list all of the possible side effects that clinical studies revealed. The medical dictionary defines a drug as "(1) a chemical substance that affects the processes of the mind or body and (2) any chemical compound used in the diagnosis, treatment, or prevention of disease or other abnormal condition."[54] As vaccines are drugs, your pediatrician should be up-to-date on the latest research about the vaccine's efficacy and possible risks—and he should share this information with you. Having to keep up with the latest medical literature, your pediatrician should be aware of the potentially life-threatening risks involved in vaccinating your child. This information is available in every package insert and on PubMed, which is comprised of more than 21 million citations for bio-medical literature from MEDLINE, life-science journals, and online books. I found this information, and certainly medical professionals have access to it as well.

Given all the scientific evidence accessible through PubMed or package inserts, parents should be able to expect a pediatrician to respond to parents' fears and anxiety with warmth, sympathy, and understanding—as the Hippocratic Oath requires. In my experience, most parents' concerns about vaccines, however, are met by a cold shoulder, hostility, and a refusal to understand. When asked by a parent whether there are any risks involved in vaccinations, most pediatricians will respond, "No more than any other medication."

This is simply not true. First, I couldn't find any package inserts for commonly used drugs like antibiotics or pain relievers that show deaths in research subjects during clinical trials. Second, while it is true that there are pos-sible side effects to any medication or drug, vaccines pose a threat of more serious short-term adverse reactions, as well as such long-term reactions as in the onset of an autoimmune disease. Third, the half-life of a commonly used medication doesn't exceed more than a short period of time, whereas vaccine adjuvants like aluminum have a half-life of over four years. More importantly it is completely unknown what damage these adjuvants do while remaining in children's organisms for such a long time.

An article on Medline states: "Up to this time, no biological function has been attributed to this metal (aluminum), and, more importantly, aluminum accumulation in tissues and organs results in their dysfunction and toxicity."[55]

The next time your doctor tells you that a vaccine is no more risky than "any other medication," ask him if the administration of one dosage of any other medication can have the same disastrous effects as the administration of aluminum.

In the next chapter I am providing you with an idea how doctors convince themselves that vaccines are effective and safe (by ignoring those studies contradicting their viewpoint) before concluding with doctors who opt not to vaccinate and their reasons for doing so.

Vaccine Research and Confirmation Bias

Confirmation bias means looking only for research supporting rather than contradicting an idea or opinion. I just read an article by Prof. Dr. Burkhard Schneeweiss and Dr. Brigitte Keller Stanislawski titled "*Vaccine Safety versus Vaccine Skepticism.*" I found this on the website of the University of Bielefeld in Germany. This article is written so convincingly and eloquently that after reading it, *I* was almost convinced that vaccines are safe—even after spending months researching vaccine safety and coming to the conclusion that vaccines are highly dangerous. This is exactly the kind of reassuring article that pediatricians fall back on and recite when addressing parental concerns, and therefore, it's worth looking at carefully to see how it works.

The authors write: "After all, millions of vaccines (including mercury and thimerosal) have been successfully used for over sixty years."[56] A concerned parent sees "millions of vaccines" and "sixty years" and thinks, *well; vaccines must be safe if they've been used successfully for such a long time, and in such large quantities.*

But where is the research proving that millions of vaccines have been used successfully for sixty years? And what exactly do the authors mean by *used successfully?*

What's their definition of *success?* They simply don't tell us.

Since we're talking about a medical procedure, however, it seems reasonable to hazard a definition of *successful* as, "effective and safe." The *Merriam-Webster Diction-ary* defines *safe* as, "not causing harm or injury; *especially* having a low incidence of adverse reactions and significant side effects when adequate instructions for use are given and having a low potential for harm under conditions of widespread availability."[57]

Are vaccines free of harm and risk? Do vaccines *not cause injury* in children? Where have vaccinated children been compared to non-vaccinated children for sixty years to establish that vaccines are indeed free of harm and risk and actually work? The fact is, no research has been conducted, and thus, the statement that millions of vaccines have been used successfully for sixty years is scientifically unsupported. Millions of vaccines have been given over the past sixty years—that much is undeniable. Also undeniable is the fact that many children have suffered immediate adverse reactions including death and permanent disability over those sixty years—clearly documented by the US government's Vaccine Adverse Event Reporting System (VAERS).

And there are other silent and long-term reactions to the vaccines that never show up on VAERS. As a matter of fact, plenty of research articles in the National Library of Medicine refute the idea that vaccine adjuvants are safe. In an article from the Neural Dynamics Research Group, Department of Ophthalmology and Visual Sciences, University of British Columbia, Vancouver, the authors write, "Immune challenges during early development, including those vaccine-induced, can lead to permanent detrimental alterations of the brain and immune function. Experimental evidence also shows that simultaneous administration of as little as two to three immune adjuvants can overcome genetic resistance to autoimmunity."[58] This means that adjuvants in every vaccine may very well cause autoimmune diseases in your child.

Then why are those adjuvants permissible? According to the researchers, it is because: "according to the US Food and Drug Administration, safety assessments for vaccines have often not included appropriate toxicity studies because vaccines have not been viewed as inherently toxic."[59] In other words: the same government agency that assures you that vaccines are safe has not studied and researched all the ingredients in those vaccines.

Therefore, pediatricians who tell you that vaccines are completely safe do so based on inappropriate or nonexistent toxicity studies. The attitude is to simply inject as many children with unknown substances and see how it affects them. In *New Developments in Vaccine Research—Unveiling the Secret of Vaccine Adjuvants,* the authors find that adjuvants in vaccines are "an ill-defined substance that non-specifically triggers the innate immune system and boosts an immune response, with aluminum-based adjuvants most commonly used in most present vaccines."[60]

In VAERS, doctors who reported adverse reactions following the hepatitis B vaccine record a wide range of symptoms. In "Autoimmunity Following Hepatitis B Vaccine as Part of the Spectrum of Autoimmune (Autoinflammatory) Syndrome Induced by Adjuvants (ASIA):

Analysis of 93 Cases," the authors conclude: "Common clinical characteristics were observed among ninety-three patients diagnosed with immune-mediated conditions post-HBV, suggesting a common denominator in these diseases."[61] J.B. Stübgen from the *Department of Neurology and Neuroscience at Weill Cornell Medical College/New York Presbyterian Hospital* admits: "Conceivably, the hepatitis B vaccines have a potential to occasionally trigger the onset of immune diseases in individuals with an underlying genetic or immunological susceptibility."[62]

Dr. Maya Ram and Dr. Yehuda Shoenfeld from the *Center for Autoimmune Diseases and Department of Medicine B, Sheba Medical Center, Tel Hashomer, Israel* conclude: "We know that the virus and vaccine share only the HBsAg (hepatitis B surface antigen) and differ in other components, and that the autoimmune response could be the consequence of different mechanisms. For example, the virus contains the DNA polymerase that was found to share an amino acid sequence with myelin basic protein, although it might trigger autoimmunity via a molecular mimicry mechanism: the vaccine, for instance, is composed of an adjuvant that might lead to the development of autoimmunity."[63]

The statement that "vaccines have been used successfully for the past sixty years" may be a comforting notion, but it's simply not true.

Doctors Who Left the Bandwagon

Most parents only see their children's pediatrician and a few other doctors routinely. They come to believe that all doctors and medical professionals share the opinion that vaccines are good and necessary. This isn't true. Many credible doctors ranging from neurosurgeons to pediatricians, as well as other health professionals ranging from nurses to professors advocate for more credible vaccine research and warn about the dangers of vaccines.

Here's what some of them have written:

- "Safety studies on vaccinations are limited to short periods. For this reason, there are valid grounds for suspecting that many delayed-type vaccine reactions may be taking place unrecognized" (Dr. Harold Buttram, FAACP, author of *Vaccines and Genetic Mutations).*

- "Vaccine trials are flawed because they aren't designed to detect associations between vaccinations and autoimmune disease," (Dr. J. Bart Classen, former researcher, National Institute of Health).

- "There is no credible scientific data to demonstrate that the injection of multiple antigens into a body is safe and effective" (Stephen C. Marini, Ph.D., Professor of Microbiology and Immunology).

- "I would challenge any colleague, clinician, or research scientist to claim we have a basic understanding of the human newborn immune system. It is well-established in studies in animal models that the newborn immune system is very distinct from the adolescent or adult. In fact, the immune system in humans can be easily perturbed to ensure it cannot respond properly in life" (Bonnie Dunbar Ph.D., Professor of Immunobiology, Baylor College of Medicine).

- "For an individual child, the risk is greater from the whooping cough vaccine than the disease" (Dr. Joanne Hatem, Medical Director, Vaccine National Information Center).

- In the *New England Journal of Medicine's* July 1994 issue, a study found that over 80% of children under five years of age who had contracted whooping cough had been fully vaccinated.

- "Dutch scientists are struggling to identify the exact cause of an epidemic of whooping cough that has swept throughout the country despite ["despite" or because of?] vaccination rates as high as 96%. Similar problems are being reported in Norway and Denmark" (*British Medical Journal*).

- "Among school-aged children, measles outbreaks have occurred in schools with vaccine levels greater than 98%. These outbreaks have occurred in all parts of the country including areas that have not reported measles for years" (*Morbidity and Mortality Weekly Report,* 2/19/89).

- There has never been a single vaccine in this country that has ever been submitted to a controlled scientific study. They never took a group of 100 people who were candidates for a vaccine, gave 50 of them a vaccine and left the other 50 alone and measured the outcome. And since that's never been done, that means if you want to be kind, you will call vaccines an unproven remedy. If you want to be accurate, you will call people who give vaccines quacks" (Robert S. Mendelsohn, M.D., Professor of Pediatrics, University of Illinois, College of Medicine).[64]

Calling a medical doctor a "quack" is a harsh word. It led me to look up the definition of "quack" in the medical dictionary. There, it is defined as, "one who misrepresents their ability and experience in diagnosis and treatment of disease or effects to be achieved by their treatment."[65] A pediatrician claiming that vaccines will prevent illness and are safe, based on no controlled scientific studies, makes unverified claims. As Dr. Mendelsohn rightfully states, with regards to vaccines' safety and effectiveness, these unverified and possibly false and unsupported claims define this pediatrician as a "quack."

The final chapters will look at the impact of a vaccine injury on an individual as well as the entire family. I will also make the case that vaccines have caused my daughters' type-1 diabetes and establish a link between vaccines and autoimmune disorders. In court it has been proven that vaccines cause autoimmune disorders. I will look at one of those cases. As more researchers come to find a causal effect of vaccines causing the immune system to turn against itself, hopefully the research community will look at reversal effects. If a vaccine has the potential of re-programming the immune system, it should be possible to reverse the effects.

Something Personal or What's at Stake

4:30 a.m. The alarm goes off. I look beside me, and my two-year-old son sleeps peacefully. I give him a kiss and get up. I grab my running shorts and socks. Then I walk across the hallway to put on my shoes and grab my suitcase. In it are my work clothes and everything else I need to get ready. Before I go downstairs, I listen at my daughter's room. My wife and daughter are still asleep. Our children have never slept alone since they were born. My son slept with my wife in a bed after his birth. This was particularly challenging when she nursed him and had to work throughout the day. She did the same for our daughter. We wanted only the best for our children. Their intellectual, physical, and emotional growth was, and is, of the utmost importance to us.

We were in the phase of transitioning our daughter to sleeping alone in her own room and bed when she was three-and-a-half years old. Then she was diagnosed with type-1 diabetes, and now her glucose levels have to be checked at night. As my wife has stayed home with the children since the diagnosis, she has taken on the task of watching over our daughter at night. I moved into the master bedroom with my son. He is two now, and I treasure every moment with him. Sometimes he curls up into my arms in the middle of the night, and my father heart enjoys this tremendously. I love my children more than anything in life. Parenthood is the toughest, most-challenging, and most-loving journey I have ever been on.

When my daughter was born four years ago, I couldn't stop crying. I am not the crying type, and I don't show emotions very often, but I will never forget that moment. I held this human, this little innocent and beautiful being in my arms, and I promised to her and God that I would always be there for her and do anything to protect her. I told her that there would never be anything more important in my life. As a native of Germany, I also promised her that I would give her the gift of two languages. I started talking to her in German and never spoke a word of English to her. By the time she was three, we had read thousands of German books and sung hundreds of German songs. She is now four, fluent in English and German, and knows the alphabet and can count in both languages. She is also a good translator. The past two years were particularly challenging as I had two children to read and sing to, play with, and be responsible for. As a father and husband, I feel it is my responsibility to teach and educate my children and spend as much time with them as possible.

It is 4:35 a.m. now, as I am heading down the stairs. This is the only time I have to run, as my time after work is reserved for my children and family. I head in the kitchen and clean the counter. Then I turn on the dishwasher so my wife can make breakfast for the children when she comes down. I pack my lunch for work and head out to the car. As I am driving to the YMCA, I am worrying about us and our family. Since my daughter was diagnosed and my wife stopped working to care for both children full time, our income has been diminished. How will we be able to survive in the future? I ask God to care for us and not let us fall and keep his hands under my family. I park the car and hit the road.

It is 5:00 a.m. on an awesome morning in March. The temperature reads 61°F, and the birds are chirping. The blooms on the trees smell beautifully, and I am running on the middle of a two-lane road. No cars are on the street yet. It is just me and the road. I am able to clear my thoughts. My legs are still mildly aching from the race on Saturday and the eight miles I ran yesterday morning. I am thinking about my book. Thinking about the responsibility I have towards others. I wonder how convinced I am. *Has my research been thorough enough to warn other parents?* I review my work and conclude that everything is as it should be. There's just a little voice in my head wondering if I should add a little something more personal.

I look at my watch. I have been running for thirty minutes, and it is time to head back. At 6:00 a.m., I finish my run after 7.2 miles. It wasn't a fast run, but a beautiful and relaxing run. I head inside the Y to clean up. At 6:15 a.m., I am in the car heading for work.

This is my fifteenth year of teaching. With the birth of my children, I have become their teacher, too. I put my life on hold completely until my daughter was three-and-a-half and my son almost two. As my work assignment changed, and the early morning time freed up, I started to workout. I transformed my body, as I believe that a healthy father is a better father. My early morning workouts and a healthier diet helped me drop from 202 pounds to 152 pounds. I feel better, and more importantly, I am a good example to my children. They see their parents eat healthily and hear us talking about our workouts and running. My daughter wants to run a race with me, and that makes me very happy.

My wife and I have been happily married for thirteen years. "Happily" doesn't mean "without challenges," but I am blessed to be married to a wife who loves me beyond my flaws. We mutually respect each other, and I am extremely happy to want to marry my wife all over again after thirteen years of marriage. Our children are lucky to have parents who, after thirteen years of marriage, love each other more every year.

When I leave work at the end of the day, I am tired—but excited by the thought of having my children around me. I am their only German-speaking encounter throughout the day, and their German will only improve and continue if I take the time. At home we will play, read, sing, and have a constant German conversation going. When the children are in bed, I mostly end up lying in my wife's lap, snoring away until she lets me know it is time to go to bed. At 4:30 a.m., the alarm will sound again

Vaccines Turning our World Upside Down

The close proximity of my daughter's multiple vaccines to her diagnosis led me on a journey of research to understand what could have possibly happened. There are also too many children affected or killed by vaccines. A little voice inside of me became louder, and I started looking at vaccines as a possible cause for my daughter's type-1 diabetes. My suspicion became stronger when I began to see the connection between the A1C tests, the timing of her multiple shots, and the onset of full-blown type-1 diabetes. At this point, this journey became inevitable. It has also been a very difficult journey, as over and over again, I've come to the conclusion that I hurt my children by having them exposed to vaccines.

I became very angry during this journey: angry at pediatricians who promote vaccination without ever having read the package inserts of the products they promote. I am angry at pediatricians who learn sound methodology in medical school, yet, seem to not have any problems when it comes to methodically unsound safety studies done by pharmaceutical companies to make parents think that vaccines are safe. I am angry at pediatricians who are being taught by and only listen to the industry-influenced AAP (American Academy of Pediatrics), FDA (Federal Drug Administration) and the CDC (Center for Disease Control) rather than thinking and researching for themselves. I am stunned to have trusted my children's pediatricians who receive almost all of their vaccine education and information from the pharmaceutical companies, who produce the material in medical school textbooks and for continuing education for doctors. I am mad and disappointed at myself for not having done more research before exposing my children to vaccines. I always heard a little voice inside me warning me about the medical intervention called immunization. This voice became apparent the first time after Johanna received her hepatitis B shot after birth in the hospital. It led me to research vaccines on the surface, but not in depth. I remember our first visit to the pediatrician. When asked about immunizing Johanna I told him that children have died right after receiving a vaccine. He looked at me and said: "Oh really?" It is a shame that the answer wasn't more like: "I know that some children have very bad side effects, including death." We put Johanna on a delayed vaccine schedule allowing only one vaccine at a time. That decision was made after I read the *Vaccine Book* by Dr. Sears. In hindsight I wish I had never come across this book and continued research on my own instead. The book basically weighs the risks as well as pros and cons of giving a vaccine. As I found out later, spreading out vaccines gives the immune system and the brain a little more time to mature; however, the assault on the immune system and the brain caused by adjuvants is just as damaging as receiving all vaccines during one office visit. This book by Dr. Sears addresses concerned parents, but doesn't provide an in-depth look into industry practices to promote vaccine safety and discuss all of the possible short term and long-term side effects. Then, when Johanna was about to start preschool, I let myself be coerced into giving her multiple vaccines in a short time period. Previously I cited a research article that states that experimental evidence shows that simultaneous administration of as few as two to three immune adjuvants can overcome genetic resistance to autoimmunity. Johanna received too many immune adjuvants in a short period of time, which I believe overexcited her little immune system and caused her immune system to turn against itself, ending in type-1 diabetes.

Diabetes Mellitus and Vaccines

Diabetes Mellitus (also type-1 diabetes or juvenile diabetes) has been around for a long time. One recent German article suggested that it might be the oldest illness known to man.

It is also extremely common today. Every hour, three children in the United States are diagnosed with type-1 diabetes.[66] However, type-1 diabetes's incidence was very low in the first half of the twentieth century. Type-1 diabetes, especially in young children, became more prevalent during the second half of the twentieth century and really began to surge during the past twenty years.[67] Researchers also see a trend in the increased prevalence of other autoimmune disorders. Not only are certain autoimmune disorders increasingly common, but the autoimmune diseases, as a class, seem to be on the rise.[68]

Personally, I am convinced that vaccines are actively making our children sick today. Not only because the rise in type-1 diabetes and other autoimmune disorders followed the increase in mass vaccinations of children at younger ages, but also because of the timeline of my daughter's diagnosis to her vaccines. In "Vaccination and Autoimmunity—*Vaccinosis:* a dangerous liaison," Shoenfeld and Aron-Maor from the Department of Internal Medicine B, Sheba Medical Center in Tel Hashomer, Israel, write:

> Even though the data regarding the relation between vaccination and autoimmune disease is conflicting, it seems that some autoimmune phenomena are clearly related to immunization…We discuss the pros and cons of this issue, although the temporal relationship (i.e., always 2–3 months following immunization) is impressive.[69]

My daughter was diagnosed with type-1 diabetes three months after she received multiple vaccines. It seems like the researchers in the above-cited article see the same timeline between vaccination and the onset of autoimmune disorder as we saw in our daughter.

After reading Tomljenovic and Shaw in "Mechanisms of Aluminum Adjuvant Toxicity and Autoimmunity in Pediatric Populations," it became obvious why I was meeting many parents of children with type-1 diabetes who couldn't find any family history of type-1 diabetes. The authors write: "Experimental evidence also shows that simultaneous administration of as little as two to three immune adjuvants can overcome genetic resistance to autoimmunity."[70]

Before mass vaccination of babies and little children occurred, autoimmune disorders such as type-1 diabetes and asthma were genetically passed on, and fewer cases were observed. Since mass-vaccinating began, we've seen much higher numbers of autoimmune diseases in younger children, because—as the researchers stated—the adjuvants found in vaccines can overcome genetic resistance and cause the immune system to turn against itself.

Our Daughter and Type-1 Diabetes

Every single decision concerning our daughter was discussed, researched, and reconsidered. She was breastfed and bathed every day. We separated vaccines to ensure that her little immune system wouldn't be challenged too much (back then I didn't understand the effects of adjuvants in vaccines). She was fed healthily, and intellectually stimulated. By the time she was three, we marveled at her. We had done everything by the book, so what could go wrong?

Well, something went unnoticed. Silently, her own immune system began to attack her pancreas, and more specifically, the insulin-producing cells in her pancreas. As her pancreas began to produce less and less insulin, her blood sugars rose and caused her to be emotionally irritable and lose weight. We took her to the doctor and then to the emergency room at Cincinnati Children's Hospital. There Johanna was diagnosed with type-1 diabetes. *What? we wondered. Diabetes? How is this possible? She isn't fat. She has always been fed healthily. She has always been an active and healthy child. How can our child have diabetes?*

Soon we learned the difference between type-1 and type-2 diabetes. We were told that type-1 diabetes can strike any child, anyone, at anytime, and has nothing to do with diet or nutrition. Type-1 diabetes is an autoimmune disorder, just like asthma. Within Johanna's immune system one or possibly both of the following scenarios happened:

1. Her B-cells produced antibodies to "flag" her insulin-producing beta cells. The "killer" T-cells, which usually only kill foreign invaders, began to destroy her insulin-producing cells.

2. Her "regulatory" T-cells did not distinguish between her own healthy cells and foreign invaders, therefore "allowing" the attack to happen.

The Adaptable Immune System (simplifed)

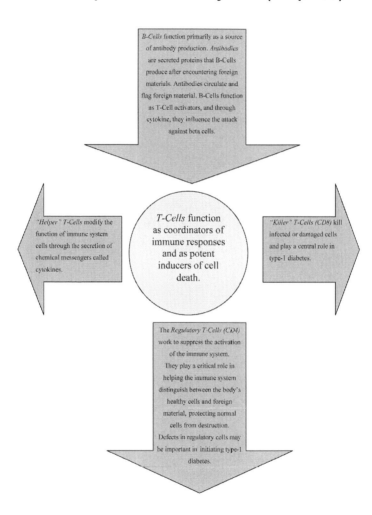

B-Cells function primarily as a source of antibody production. *Antibodies* are secreted proteins that B-Cells produce after encountering foreign materials. Antibodies circulate and flag foreign material. B-Cells function as T-Cell activators, and through cytokine, they influence the attack against beta cells.

T-Cells function as coordinators of immune responses and as potent inducers of cell death.

"Helper" T-Cells modify the function of immune system cells through the secretion of chemical messengers called cytokines.

"Killer" T-Cells (CD8) kill infected or damaged cells and play a central role in type-1 diabetes.

The *Regulatory T-Cells (CD4)* work to suppress the activation of the immune system. They play a critical role in helping the immune system distinguish between the body's healthy cells and foreign material, protecting normal cells from destruction. Defects in regulatory cells may be important in initiating type-1 diabetes.

Regulatory T-Cells play a critical role in protecting the body's own cells, such as the insulin-producing cells, from being attacked by the body's own immune system. When we look at how vaccines work, it is fairly obvious that there has to be a connection between immunization and the development of type-1 diabetes. The antibodies secreted by B-cells circulate throughout the human body and attack the microbes that have not yet infected any cells but are lurking in the blood or the spaces between cells. When antibodies gather on the surface of a microbe, it becomes unable to function. Antibodies signal macrophages and other defensive cells to come eat the microbe. Antibodies also work with other defensive molecules that circulate in the blood, called complement proteins, to destroy microbes. The work of B-cells is called the humoral immune response, or simply the antibody response. The goal of most vaccines is to stimulate this response. In reality, many infectious microbes can be defeated by antibodies alone, without any help from killer T-cells."[71] Vaccines, however, are designed to stimulate B-cells or B-cell functioning. B-cells produce the antibodies needed to attack insulin-producing cells.

> In 1991, the Italian government implemented a mandatory hepatitis B immunization program, requiring all children to receive the vaccine when they either reached three months or twelve years of age. No vaccinations were given at any other age to people in the study, and no catch-up vaccination program was implemented for children between those ages. In their study, the scien-

tists measured the incidence of type-I diabetes in vaccinated and unvaccinated children from central Italy. They also measured the differences related to their ages at the times they were vaccinated. The overall relative risk of type I diabetes in vaccinated versus unvaccinated children was 1.34. This means that any children who received the hepatitis B vaccine would be 34% more likely to develop diabetes than unvaccinated children. While this overall risk of diabetes may not seem that great, the statistics took a dramatic increase in children who were vaccinated at age twelve. In that group, the relative risk was measured at 2.58. In other words, children who received the hepatitis B vaccine at age twelve were more than 2.5 times as likely to be diagnosed with type I diabetes as their unvaccinated peers. Based on their findings, the scientists concluded that children inoculated with the hepatitis B vaccine are at an increased risk of type I diabetes. They also suggested that "hepatitis B vaccine per se, or the timing of administration, must be reconsidered to reduce the risk associated with it" (Pozzilli P, et al. "Hepatitis B Vaccine Associated with an Increased Type I Diabetes in Italy." Presented at the annual meeting of the American Diabetes Association, San Antonio, TX, June 13, 2000).

Several large studies conducted in the 1990s have provided convincing evidence that vaccines may be associated with the development of type-1 diabetes. In New Zealand in 1996, researchers saw a 60% increase in childhood diabetes cases after the country had a mass hepatitis B vaccination campaign from 1988 to 1991 for infants six weeks and older. Finland has had a vaccination programs for decades, and J. Barthelow Claasen, M.D., a former researcher at the National Institute of Health, has been documenting a vaccine-diabetes connection. In *Infectious Disease in Clinical Practice,* he reported that the incidence of diabetes in Finland was stable in children younger than four years of age until the government modified its immunization schedule. In 1974 a total of 130,000 children aged three months to four years received HIB or meningitis vaccine. In 1976, the government added a second pertussis strain to its pertussis vaccine. Between 1977 and 1979, the incidence of type-1 diabetes increased by 64% compared to 1970 to 1976. Overall, childhood diabetes increased by 147% in children younger than three years after all the vaccine changes were made (Cave, Stephanie, M.D.; Mitchell, Deborah. *What Your Doctor May Not Tell You about Children's Vaccinations,* Google Books, 2001).

New Reality

Here we are. Our lives, and most importantly, the life of our three-year-old daughter has changed forever. There is *no* cure. This isn't a contagious disease, but it is extremely challenging for everyone to manage it. As Johanna's little body doesn't produce insulin, she has to get a shot after every meal. The injected insulin keeps her alive and hopefully free of long-term complications; however, insulin by injection can also be extremely dangerous, as it can lead to hypoglycemia, or low blood sugar, which will cause shaking, seizures, and even death if undetected. To avoid high blood sugar, she needs more insulin, and she has to be corrected by injection. In order to detect both, we have to check her blood sugar day and night, pricking her and taking a small blood sample. There is much more to managing this illness, but in a nutshell, this is what we are facing.

What I wish the most? That I had known about type-1 diabetes and vaccines before Johanna was vaccinated. I wish that as a parent, I would have known that this illness could strike my child, no matter how well I took care of her. I wish I had known that vaccines (or adjuvants in vaccines) have been implicated to cause autoimmune disorders.

Why wasn't I told by Johanna's pediatrician? Had I known about it, I would have done some things differently. I would have been more responsible and skeptical, not letting the government and health officials scare me into vaccinating my children. Hindsight is 20/20 vision, and the research journey I embarked on painted a clearer picture as to all that I could have done—or *not* done. I would not have vaccinated my child.

According to most epidemiologists, at present, research on what triggers type-1 diabetes is inconclusive. Basically, any child can be struck at any time. Personally I think they are mistaken. If more scientists would research the link between vaccine adjuvants and auto-immune disorders, they would find that vaccines cause autoimmune disorders and chronic illnesses in children. However, according to some in the scientific community there are other correlations, other factors that could possibly cause or trigger type-1 diabetes:

Genetics

Researchers believe that genetics play a role. However, it is commonly believed that genetic predisposition and environmental factors have to intertwine to trigger type-1 diabetes. A person can live with a genetic predisposition all his or her life and never get the disease if that person is never exposed to the environmental triggers. However, some of the research I have cited suggests that vaccines can overcome genetic resistance, causing the immune system of people without genetic predisposition towards type-1 diabetes to "change its thinking."

Environmental Factors

Studies are inconclusive, but some researchers believe that cow's milk could be a trigger. Other studies suggest good hygiene (meaning too many baths and not enough exposure to viruses and bacteria) could be a trigger, as the immune system isn't challenged enough, and is therefore underdeveloped. Researchers are also very interested in viral infections (particularly coxsackie B virus, mumps, and rubella).

Researching environmental links to type-1 diabetes is certainly important to and for people who develop type-1 diabetes but have never received vaccines. However, as vaccine adjuvants can overcome genetic resistance the importance of studying the vaccinated population suffering from autoimmune disorders is equally important.

Vaccines

Correlation studies conducted in Italy and New Zealand show a correlation of the introduction of the hepatitis B vaccine and increases in type-1 diabetes. Another study conducted in Italy shows a significant link between type-1 diabetes incidence and mumps and rubella. The MMR vaccine given is a live-vaccine; therefore, children are exposed to a live mumps and rubella virus. Other correlation studies suggest a link between type-1 diabetes and certain vaccines. "As early as 1949, the medical literature reported that some people injected with the pertussis vaccine had reduced glucose levels. The pertussis vaccine can also cause diabetes in mice. In 1997, US federal health officials did admit that one of their own studies showed that the possibility that hepatitis B vaccinations, particularly at older ages, may increase patients' risk for type-1 diabetes cannot be ruled out and will require larger detailed studies." To date, however, I have been unable to discover where, or whether the "larger detailed studies" have been conducted.

A statement of research scientist Dr. Bonnie Dunbar to the Immunization Division at the Texas Department of Health made me focus more on vaccine safety and particularly on the hepatitis B vaccine:

> I was honored a few years ago by the National Institutes of Health in Washington D.C. as the "First Margaret Pittman" lecturer for my pioneering work in vaccine development. This was a most special event for me because of Dr. Pittman's contributions to early vaccines and because I understand the impact that some vaccines have had (and will continue to have) on our society. My ongoing research in the area of vaccine development continues to be a major commitment. I have worked extensively with the US Agency for International Development and the World Health Organization programs and have a lifelong commitment to carrying our research to understand, and hopefully, help to solve world population as well as disease problems.
>
> I am speaking to you today, however, in reference to my experience with the severe adverse effects of the hepatitis B vaccine. About five years ago, I had two individuals working in my laboratory who were required to take the hepatitis B vaccine. Both of these individuals developed severe and apparently permanent adverse reactions as a result of this vaccine. Both of these individuals were completely healthy and very athletic before this vaccine, and have now suffered severe,

debilitating autoimmune side effects from this vaccine. I know the complete medical history of one, Dr. Bohn Dunbar...my brother, who developed serious rashes, joint pain, chronic fatigue, multiple sclerosis-like symptoms, and now, has been affirmatively diagnosed with POTS (an autoimmune cardiovascular neurological problem) and finally with chronic inflammatory demyelinating polyneuropathy. His problems have been attributed to the hepatitis B vaccine by over a dozen different specialists around the United States of unquestionable medical expertise. He has now been rated permanently and totally impaired at greater than 90%. His health care has already cost the state of Texas around a half-million dollars in the Worker's Compensation Program to date, a figure that will continue to rise given the severity of his health condition.

My other student went partially blind following her first booster injection, a medical condition that was markedly exacerbated by her second booster, which resulted in long-term hospitalization. Personal communications are that her eyesight is continuing to deteriorate. Because she is in medical school, she has been (understandably so) afraid to pursue investigation into her medical problems in the event that they might affect her medical career.

As I have worked extensively in vaccine development, I am extremely sensitive to the need to evaluate the risk vs. benefits of any vaccine. Because of my established expertise in this area, it became immediately apparent to me that these two active, healthy individuals working in my laboratory developed "autoimmune" syndromes at a predictable immunological time frame following their booster injections to the hepatitis B vaccine. After carrying out extensive literature research on this vaccine, it became immediately apparent that the serious adverse side effects of this vaccine (which appear to be related to the nature of the viral protein itself), may be more significant than generally known.[73]

Johanna and Multiple Vaccines – From Insult to Injury

Johanna received one hepatitis B vaccine at birth. Then we allowed for only one shot at a time until Johanna was two years old. After I started researching vaccines, we held off on vaccines until she started pre-school. As the state of Kentucky mandates vaccinations, and our pediatricians politely let us know that if we did not give Johanna the MMR vaccine, they wouldn't allow her in the office, I felt compelled to agree to have her injected with more vaccines. At that point, I also hadn't done extensive research on vaccines. Johanna received her MMR vaccine on April 22, 2011, her second hepatitis B shot on June 15, 2011, her third hepatitis B shot on August 10, 2011 and her PCV13 vaccine in August 22, 2011. Ten days after her MMR vaccine she developed a severe rash all over her body. A few weeks after her second hepatitis B shot she started to become more emotionally irritable. A few days after her PCV13 shot she developed red hives covering almost every body part. She was diagnosed with type-1 diabetes at Cincinnati Children's Hospital on September 27, 2011.

When Johanna was hospitalized, an A1C blood test was conducted. What is the A1C test? This test measures excess sugar in the blood. It is a test that can "look back." Here is more specifically how the A1C test works:

Hemoglobin, a protein that links up with sugars such as glucose, is found inside red blood cells. Its job is to carry oxygen from the lungs to all the cells of the body. When diabetes is uncontrolled, you end up with too much glucose in the bloodstream. This extra glucose enters your red blood cells and links up (or glycates) with molecules of hemoglobin. The more excess glucose in your blood, the more hemoglobin gets glycated. By measuring the percentage of A1C in the blood, you get an overview of your average blood glucose control for the past few months.[74]

As Johanna's insulin-producing cells were killed off by her own immune system, more excess glucose circulated in her bloodstream. Without the needed insulin in her body, there was no way for the glucose to be transported to her cells in order to get energy. Her body then began to break down fatty tissue for energy, which caused her to lose weight and be extremely thirsty. Here is where the A1C test comes in. The test measures her excess glucose over her past three months; however, 50% of the test results account for the last months before measurement. Johanna began receiving multiple shots approximately three months before we saw symptoms. Something in those vaccines caused her B-cells or T-cells to be misdirected and turn against her own insulin-producing beta cells. As beta cells were being killed slowly, we couldn't see any symptoms in the first eight weeks after vaccinations. Her pancreas still produced insulin. With only a few beta cells left, we began to see symptoms. Thanks to the A1C test, we were able to look back three months, and thanks to the recording of her vaccinations, we can clearly see how the onset of diabetes and vaccination correlate.

Johanna did not suffer from any other virus or bacterial infection during this time except for the vaccine induced rashes prior to onset of symptoms. It is commonly understood that whence type-1 diabetes is triggered, it progresses gradually and quickly until the first symptoms are noticeable. The general consensus is that it takes a few months from the moment the disease is triggered to the onset of symptoms when most of the body's beta cells have been destroyed. The A1C test showed high glucose levels beginning approximately June 15 with the highest levels beginning approximately August 15 as the insulin production in Johanna's body came to an end. As Johanna didn't show any symptoms of a viral or bacterial infection, the MMR vaccine is the only live virus Johanna was injected with. How then could vaccines cause type-1 diabetes? I began to wonder if there have been other people with an autoimmune disease onset three months after receiving vaccines.

More about the Hepatitis B Vaccine

In 1999, nurse Patti White testified before the US Congress. Parts of her testimony included the following:

> "For the past three or four years our school district has noted a significant increase in the number of children entering school with developmental disorders, learning disabilities, attention deficit disorders and/or serious chronic illness such as diabetes, asthma and seizure disorders. Each of the past four years has been worse than the year before. There is only one common thread we have been able to identify in these children: they are the children who received the first trial hepatitis B injections as newborns in the early 1990s. As the hepatitis B compliance rate in newborns has gone up in our community, so has the percentage of damaged children. This is very alarming. Because of having so many damaged children we have tried to find the long-term clinical trials that ruled this vaccine "safe and effective." We discovered through an exhaustive Medline search that the FDA based its decision to approve hepatitis B vaccine for administration in the first hours of a newborn baby's life upon clinical trials and upon post-marketing surveillance studies in which patients and their doctors were asked to report any adverse effects they noticed within 4-5 days after each injection [4 days for SmithKline and 5 days for Merck]."[75]

Most important to me is that *our government approves drugs to be injected into our children without having conducted exhaustive studies on possible side effects*.

The next part of Patti White's testimony struck home with me, as it is directly linked to what happened to my daughter. She said,

> The problems being reported in increasing numbers as occurring after hepatitis B vaccination appear to be autoimmune and neurological in origin. Such problems take weeks to months to produce noticeable symptoms, and cannot be spotted in a 4-5 day observation period. These are the only clinical studies that have been done by Merck or SmithKline. There is not one long-term study that we could find."[76]

Not only this correlation alone, but the testimonies of many others I have found make me think that this vaccine could be the culprit in causing my child to suffer from type-1 diabetes.

I now better understand doctors and nurses who advocated that my child be immunized. As nurse Patty, who has worked twenty-five years as nurse, said: "I have repeated the well-rehearsed refrain, 'Be Wise; Immunize,' thousands of times during those years, and reassured countless parents that they were doing the right thing by vaccinating their precious children...even the ones who came to me with serious doubts and reservations. I will now have to live with that." And furthermore: " I personally have had to research this on my own to determine if I have been enforcing a policy that is actually harming more children than it will ever help. I have spent countless hours reading books, vaccine-hearing testimony, research papers, medical journal articles, and Internet Web sites from around the world. I did not come to my decision easily or lightly, I assure you. Twenty-five years of total belief in something does not shake that easily."[77]

Most doctors and nurses, who will tell you and told me that vaccines are safe, have never researched vaccines and vaccine safety. They are simply reciting what they have learned in nursing school or medical school. Those who started thinking for themselves and conducting extensive personal research often come to different conclusions.

Mr. Belkin came to this different conclusion. In his testimony before the Advisory Committee on Immunization Practices at the Center for Disease Control, he explains why: "My daughter, Lyla Rose Belkin, died on September 16, 1998, at the age of five weeks, shortly after receiving her hepatitis B vaccine booster shot."[78]

In his search for answers, Mr. Belkin attended a hepatitis B vaccine workshop at the National Academy of Science. The workshop hosted doctors and scientists from all across the United States and Europe. Later, he testified to Congress about what he witnessed at that workshop:

> The presentations included a study of Animal Models of Newborn Responses to Antigen

Presentation, which showed that newborn immune systems were underdeveloped and strikingly different than those of adults. The message I received was that immune response in a newborn to shocks such as being injected with a vaccine was potentially unknown, since newborn T-Cells have radically different behavior than those of adults. Another presentation was "Strategies for Evaluating the Biologic Mechanisms of Hepatitis B Vaccine Reactions," in which vaccine researcher Dr. Bonnie Dunbar of Baylor College related numerous hepatitis B-vaccine-related cases of nervous system damage in adults, such as multiple sclerosis, seizures, and blindness. On the more positive side, the FDA (Federal Drug Administration) presented a seemingly reassuring study from its Vaccine Adverse Events Reporting System (VAERS), which showed only nineteen neonatal deaths reported since 1991 related to hepatitis B vaccination.[79]

Correlation versus Causality

Looking for more correlative evidence that linked vaccines to autoimmune disorders, I came across: DOROTHY WERDERITSH, v. SECRETARY OF HEALTH AND HUMAN SERVICES (99-319V), Date Filed: 05/26/2006, Case Number:

99-319V, Entitlement; Hepatitis B vaccine and multiple sclerosis.

The discussion section of the publication states:

This is causation in fact case. To satisfy her burden of proving causation in fact,

> petitioner must offer "(1) a medical theory causally connecting the vaccination and the injury; (2) a logical sequence of cause and effect showing that the vaccination was the reason for the injury; and (3) a showing of a proximate temporal relationship between vaccination and injury." Althen v. Secretary of HHS, 418 F. 3d 1274, 1278 (Fed. Cir. 2005).

The court documents show that:

> Petitioner has shown a medical theory causally connecting the vaccination and the injury, a logical sequence of cause and effect showing the vaccine caused her injury and a proximate temporal relationship between her vaccinations and injury through the testimony of both sides' witnesses, the facts elicited from the medical

records, and the medical literature. Petitioner has prevailed in proving that hepatitis B vaccination caused or significantly aggravated her MS.[80]

In this case, the courts decided that the hepatitis B vaccine caused multiple sclerosis. The petitioner was entitled to reasonable compensation.

Molecular Mimicry

Most interesting to me wasn't the outcome of the above-mentioned case, but the medical evidence produced to prove that the hepatitis B vaccine caused multiple sclerosis. Multiple sclerosis is an autoimmune disorder just as type-1 diabetes is an autoimmune disorder. One article cited to prove that the hepatitis B vaccine caused MS in this person states:

> The authors studied a patient who developed MS three months after hepatitis B vaccination. They found cross-recognition of hepatitis B surface antigen and a proteolipid protein—derived peptide by a T-cell line isolated from the patients peripheral blood. These preliminary findings suggest to the authors that molecular mimicry might trigger autoimmune demyelination after hepatitis B vaccination.[81]

The definition of molecular mimicry was also stated in the court documents: "Molecular mimicry is the process by which T-cell activated in response to determinants on an infecting microorganism cross-react with self-epitopes, leading to an autoimmune disease".[82]

Does an Autoimmune Vaccine Cause an Autoimmune Disease?

In *Multiple Sclerosis and Hepatitis B Vaccination: Adding the Credibility of Molecular Biology to an Unusual Level of Clinical and Epidemiological Evidence,* the authors write: "A number of convergent facts, however, suggests that the manufacturing process could introduce HBV (hepatitis B vaccine) polymerase as a contaminant, and then trigger an autoimmune process against myelin in some vaccinated subjects. Of great significance, this hypothesis is likely to give the missing link to account for the considerable body of clinical and epidemiological evidence documenting that, for a drug used with a preventive purpose, HBV has an unusual potential to induce central neurological disorders amongst other unwanted side-effects."[83] Furthermore, the authors list two categories of HBV (hepatitis B-vaccine)-related side effects:

> (1) disorders reproducing almost the whole spectrum of nonhepatic manifestations of natural hepatitis B (including peripheral demyelinating disorders such as Guillain-Barre´ syndromes), generally within a quite evocative latency period (a few days or weeks)

> (2) central demyelinating disorders such as multiple sclerosis (MS), which may have their first clinical manifestations some years after vaccination.[84]

Zuckerman, in an article from 1972 in *Nature,* entitled "Hepatitis B Vaccine: A Note of Caution," pointed out "that autoimmunity might well follow the hepatitis B vaccinations because the disease, itself, involved autoimmunity" (255:104–5). One form of hepatitis B is autoimmune hepatitis B. In autoimmune hepatitis B, the body's immune system attacks the cells of the liver, just like in type-1 diabetes, where the body's immune system attacks the beta cells of the pancreas. I am confident that research in this area will confirm that the hepatitis B vaccine has the potential of causing type-1 diabetes in children and adults.

The End

Having done a lot of research, I am fully aware of the dangers vaccines pose to my children. My wife, however, felt that vaccines might actually protect our children. As my wife is a fairly emotional and spiritual person, the cold, hard scientific facts implicating vaccine dangers didn't appeal to her as much as a very personal experience. When my wife was still working, she had a flexible spending account provided by her health insurance. With that account came the responsibility to send proof of treatment to the insurance company. As my wife is staying home since our daughter's diagnosis, we still get requests from her former health insurance to provide evidence of treatment. Recently, she received a letter asking to provide proof of treatment for three dates in 2011. When she received the receipts from our pediatrician, they read in the following order:

> April 2011—MMR Vaccine
>
> May 2011— Rash
>
> September 2011—Type-1 Diabetes Diagnosis

My wife believes in signs from above, and this is all it took to convince her of the vaccine—autoimmune disease connection. That's all it took for her to be convinced of vaccines' dangers.

It took me months of research looking at various sources from various experts to finally be convinced that vaccines are not in the best interest of our children.

Besides the scientific facts and personal stories I've provided for you, I hope that more light will be shed on the damage that vaccines do. The vaccination bandwagon continues to roll through this country and the rest of the world. As children continue to be damaged by vaccines, we will not see a change in vaccine research unless more people get off the bandwagon. I wish I had read this book before immunizing my own children; I am convinced that if I had, my daughter would have been spared an autoimmune disease. My children will not receive any further vaccines until methodologically sound studies show that vaccines are safe and actually protect from illness.

How to Talk to Your Children's Doctor

You're taking your children to see their pediatrician. You've heard about the controversies surrounding vaccinations, and you start wondering whether what is being injected into your healthy children is actually good for them. You are in a small room waiting for your pediatrician, planning on discussing vaccine safety with him. You may be a little bit nervous, as you know you are up against a health professional who has been trained to convince you that immunizations are necessary for your child.

Based on my personal experience, there are several responses you may elicit from your pediatrician. You may have the following experiences:

You may encounter a very friendly doctor, who will explain to you that he has seen vaccine-preventable diseases kill children within six hours. This scares you to the core of your parental instincts. Your pediatrician shows nothing but respect for you, and genuinely seems to have your child's best interest at heart. Most parents' argument ends here, and the injections begin.

Unfortunately, your pediatrician has failed to warn you about the full scope of dangers that vaccines pose to your child. He also will not take responsibility should your child be left with a vaccine-related injury or vaccine-induced illness.

You may also encounter the friendly pediatrician who immediately rises to the challenge, verbally providing you with the results of numerous scientific and medical studies, all of which show that vaccines are not only safe for your child, but that they prevent diseases. Again, most parents' objections end here as well. And why shouldn't they? After all, scientific literature *clearly shows* that vaccines won't hurt, but will definitely help their children!

Or do they? During a conversation with a pediatrician, I mentioned my research using the National Library of Medicine and all the credible work I had found there suggesting that vaccines pose immediate as well as delayed dangers to children. She responded by pointing out that both parties, pro-vaccine and anti-vaccine, can find credible research to support their points of view.

She's right about that. However, the fact that tens of thousands of children a year experience severe reactions to vaccines puts the burden of proof firmly on the pro-vaccine side. Before we inject healthy children with toxic substances, the only studies we should be able to find are those showing, beyond a reasonable doubt, that vaccines are safe and actually work.

There is another important aspect: When your friendly and science-oriented pediatrician recites the research literature, keep one thing in mind: This research proves nothing. As I have stated already, there is no single, controlled clinical study proving that vaccines actually work. Your doctor may well pull out a package insert from the vaccine and show you the clinical studies produced by the pharmaceutical company. Read carefully and you'll find that the vaccines weren't tested against a true placebo, and that even during these studies, children died from the vaccine.

What you want to know before your child is injected with a vaccine is that, beyond a reasonable doubt, the vaccine prevents the disease your child is being vaccinated against and that the vaccine is safe. There is no scientific study out there easing your mind regarding vaccine effectiveness and safety.

You may also encounter your "risk-versus-benefit" and "you have to have faith" pediatrician. Well, again, your pediatrician will tell you that she has seen children die from vaccine-preventable illnesses, and that since the introduction of vaccines, those illnesses have declined greatly. Unfortunately, the pediatrician will say, because of a few irresponsible parents, there are still children contracting and dying from these diseases.

What can you say now? *It's true;* you may think, *there are always risks involved in life. Why would vaccines be any different?*

Vaccines are different because they are *medical interventions given to healthy individuals.* Should your child be hurt from a vaccine, you have given permission for this to happen, based on the notion that your child *may* contract a disease.

Your pediatrician's claims about the reasons for the persistence of certain diseases aren't supported by research. Nor has he mentioned the fact that more children experience vaccine-induced illnesses and side effects than contract the diseases the vaccines try to prevent. In fact, the very reason that some of these diseases persist is not because some kids don't get vaccinated. Rather, it's just the opposite: They contract the disease *because* they've been vaccinated against it.

As I have quoted in this book, the only cases of polio in this country are vaccine-induced polio cases. Children do not contract polio naturally anymore. Your pediatrician may argue that the reason why children do not contract polio naturally anymore is because of vaccines, but there also is no scientific proof behind this argument. In fact, studies have shown that most diseases were on the decline before the introduction of vaccines.

So do the benefits of immunizations really outweigh the risks? It is not at all clear that they do. Government databases show that tens of thousands suffer vaccine injuries every year; no scientific studies prove that vaccines work; and a multitude of scientific studies suggest that they *don't* work. The undeniable risks far outweigh vaccines' unsubstantiated benefits.

Another type you may encounter is the "no-tolerance" pediatrician, who will threaten to refuse seeing your children if you do not consent to having them vaccinated. Again, you have no way to argue your point.

The possible scenarios I have given above may seem to make it impossible for you to argue your point and protect your child. However, this book has provided you with more arguments to help you carry on an informed dialogue with your pediatrician. If you continue to sense that your opinion isn't being taken seriously, or if you are threatened with being refused service, rest assured, there are pediatricians in your vicinity who will work with you.

End Notes

1) "7 Signs of a Bad Doctor." *BabyCenter*. Web. 14 May 2012. <http://www.babycenter.com/0_7-signs-of-a-bad-doctor_10341016.bc?page=2>.

2) "About Us." *The Cochrane Collaboration*. Web. 14 May 2012. <http://www.cochrane.org/about-us>.

3) Adams, Mike. "Evidence-based Vaccinations: A Scientific Look at the Missing Science behind Flu Season Vaccines." *Naturalnews.com*. Web. 14 May 2012. <http://www.naturalnews.com/029641_vaccines_junk_science.html>.

4) Adams, Mike. "Merck Vaccine Scientist Dr. Maurice Hilleman Admitted Presence of SV40, AIDS, and Cancer Viruses in Vaccines." *Naturalnews.com*. Web. 14 May 2012. <http://www.naturalnews.com/033584_Dr_Maurice_Hilleman_SV40.html>.

5) "Aluminum Toxicity." *Aluminum Toxicity*. Web. 14 May 2012. <http://emedicine.medscape.com/article/165315-overview>.

6) Belkin, Michael. "Hepatitis B Vaccines: Adverse Reactions. Think Twice!" *Hepatitis B Vaccines: Adverse Reactions*. Web. 14 May 2012. <http://thinktwice.com/hepb.htm>.

7) Blaylock, Russel L. "Propaganda for Vaccine Manufacturers." *Amazon.com: Profile for Russell L. Blaylock: Reviews*. Web. 14 May 2012. <http://www.

amazon.com/gp/cdp/member-reviews/A3TBYAX-CH6YLSR/ref=cm_pdp_rev_more?ie=UTF8>.

8) Braun, Miles M. "Vaccine Adverse Event Reporting System (VAERS) - Usefulness and Limitations." *Institute for Vaccine Safety.*Web.1 July 2012. <http://www.vaccinesafety.edu/VAERS.htm>.

9) Buttram, Harold. "Safe and Effective: Fact or Fiction?" *Vaccines Uncensored*. Web. 16 May 2012. <http://www.vaccinesuncensored.org/safety.php>.

10) Centers for Disease Control and Prevention. *Centers for Disease Control and Prevention,* 08 February 2011. Web. 14 May 2012. <http://www.cdc.gov/vaccinesafety/Activities/vaers.html>.

11) Colebeck, Christine. "Death by Lethal Vaccine Infection." *Rense.com*. 17 Sept. 2004. Web. 14 May 2012. <http://www.rense.com/>.

12) Commenge, Yannik. "Multiple Sclerosis and Hepatitis B Vaccination: Adding the Credibility of Molecular Biology to an Unusual Level of Clinical and Epidemiological Evidence." *Elsevier*. Web. <http://www.vacinfo.org/MS-HepB.pdf>.

13) Janak, Cynthia A. "VAERS Reporting —Is It Accurate?" *VAERS Reporting*. Web. 14 May 2012. <http://www.renewamerica.com/columns/janak/080330>.

14) "Definition of "Quack'" *Dorland's Medical Dictionary*. Web. 16 May 2012. <http://medical-dictionary.thefreedictionary.com/quack>.

15) De Veer, M. "New Developments in Vaccine Research—Unveiling the Secret of Vaccine Adjuvants." *National Center for Biotechnology Information.* US National Library of Medicine. Web. 14 May 2012. <http://www.ncbi.nlm.nih.gov/pubmed/21955847>.

16) "Doctor of Vaccine Profit." *Child Health Safety. com.* Ed. ChildHealthSafety. Web. 14 May 2012. <http://childhealthsafety.wordpress.com/2011/04/23/ offit-congressional-reprimand/>.

17) Dunbar, Bonnie S. "Hepatitis B Vaccine." *Hepatitis B Vaccine.* Web. 14 May 2012. <http://www.gulfwarvets.com/dunbar.htm>.

18) Geier, D.A. "A Case-control Study of Serious Autoimmune Adverse Events following Hepatitis B Immunization." *National Center for Biotechnology Information.* US National Library of Medicine. Web. 15 May 2012. <http://www.ncbi.nlm.nih.gov/ pubmed/16206512>.

19) "Gesundheitliche Aufklärung." *Impfen Macht Krank.* Web. 14 May 2012. <http://www.gesundheitlicheaufklaerung.de/impfen-macht-krank>.

20) Gran, B. et.al. "Development of Multiple Sclerosis after Hepatitis B Vaccination: An Immunologic Case Report." *54 Neurology Supp. 3: 164* (2000).

21) "Haemophilus B Conjugate (Meningococcal Protein Conjugate) and Hepatitis B (Recombinant) Vaccine." Web. <http://www.merck.com/product/usa/ pi_circulars/c/comvax/comvax_pi.pdf>.

22) "Haemophilus B Conjugate Vaccine." Web. <https://www.vaccineshoppe.com/image.cfm?doc_id=11167&image_type=product_pdf>.

23) "Healthsentinel.com." *Healthsentinel.com*. Web. 14 May 2012. <http://www.healthsentinel.com/>.

24) "How Vaccines Work." *National Institute of Allergy and Infectious Disease*. Web. 14 May 2012. <http://www.niaid.nih.gov/topics/vaccines/understanding/pages/howwork.aspx>.

25) "Immunization Science." *Demographics of Unvaccinated Children*. Web. 14 May 2012. <http://www.immunizationinfo.org/science/demographics-unvaccinated-children>.

26) Karali, Z. "Autoimmunity and Hepatitis A Vaccine in Children." *National Center for Biotechnology Information*. US National Library of Medicine. Web. 15 May 2012. <http://www.ncbi.nlm.nih.gov/pubmed/21905502>.

27) Kögel-Schauz, Andrea. "Ungeimpfte Kinder Sind Gesünder." *Eltern Für Impfaufklärung*. Web. <http://www.efi-online.de/PDF/UngeimpfteGesuender.pdf>.

28) Krawitt, EL. „Patient Information: Autoimmune Hepatitis (Beyond the Basics)." *Autoimmune Hepatitis (Beyond the Basics)*. Web. 14 May 2012. <http://www.uptodate.com/contents/patient-information-autoimmune-hepatitis>.

29) Lisa. "How Do Scientists Know a Vaccine Is Safe?" *Yahoo Answers*. Web. <http://answers.yahoo.

com/question/index?qid=20100517011013AAIR
0UK>.

30) "Little Ben Trust." *Little Ben Trust*. Web. 14 May 2012. <http://www.littlebentrust.com/index.html>.

31) "Living with Diabetes." *A1C*. Web. 14 May 2012. <http://www.diabetes.org/living-with-diabetes/treatment-and-care/blood-glucose-control/a1c/>.

32) Marichal, Thomas. "DNA Released from Dying Host Cells Mediates Aluminum Adjuvant Activity." *Nature Medicine*. Web. <http://www.nature.com/nm/journal/v17/n8/full/nm.2403.html>.

33) Maya, Ram. "Hepatitis B: Infection, Vaccination, and Autoimmunity." Web. <http://www.ima.org.il/imaj/ar08jan-16.pdf>.

34) Mercola, Joseph. "60 Lab Studies Now Confirm Cancer Link to a Vaccine You Probably Had as a Child." *Mercola.com*. Web. <http://articles.mercola.com/sites/articles/archive/2011/02/18/leading-vaccine-doctor-states-cancer-linked-to-polio-vaccine.aspx>.

35) Mercola, Joseph. "Do Flu Vaccines Work?" *WeeksMD Â»*. Web. 14 May 2012. <http://weeksmd.com/2009/09/do-flu-vaccines-work/>.

36) Meroni, P.L. "Autoimmune or Auto-inflammatory Syndrome Induced by Adjuvants (ASIA): Old Truths and a New Syndrome?" *National Center for Biotechnology Information*. US National Library of Medicine. Web. 15 May 2012. <http://www.ncbi.nlm.nih.gov/pubmed/21051205>.

37) *Merriam-Webster*. Web. 14 May 2012. <http://www.merriamwebster.com/medical/safe>.

38) Miller, Neil. "Safe and Effective: Fact or Fiction?" *Vaccines Uncensored*. Web. 14 May 2012. <http://www.vaccinesuncensored.org/safety.php>.

39) Nakazawa, Donna J. "The Autoimmune Epidemic: Bodies Gone Haywire in a World Out of Balance." *Personal Health*. Web. 14 May 2012. <http://www.alternet.org/health/80129>.

40) Olson, Julie K., Eager, Todd N. and Miller, Stephen D., "Functional Activation of myelin-specific T-cells by virus induced molecular mimicry", *Journal of Immunology, 2002; 169:2719-2726.*

41) "Poliovirus Vaccine Inactivated." Web. <https://www.vaccineshoppe.com/image.cfm?doc_id=5984&image_type=product_pdf>.

42) "Prevalence and Incidence of Type 1 Diabetes." *RightDiagnosis.com*. Web. 14 May 2012. <http://www.rightdiagnosis.com/d/diab1/prevalence.htm>.

43) Rota, J.S. "Two Case Studies of Modified Measles in Vaccinated Physicians Exposed to Primary Measles Cases: High Risk of Infection but Low Risk of Transmission." *National Center for Biotechnology Information*. US National Library of Medicine. Web. 14 May 2012. <http://www.ncbi.nlm.nih.gov/pubmed/21666213>.

44) "RotaTeq Oral Solution." *Merck.com*. Web. <http://www.merck.com/product/usa/pi_circulars/r/rotateq/rotateq_pi.pdf>.

45) Schneeweiss, Burkhard. "Impfrisiken Und Impf-skepsis." *Fakultät Für Gesundheitswissenschaften.* Web. <http://www.unibielefeld.de/gesundhw/ag2/infepi/impfungen.html>.

46) Sellers, Kal. „Vaccinations: How to Recover." *Vaccinations: How to Recover.* Web. 14 May 2012. <http://www.naturalnews.com/028000_vaccinations_health_problems.html>.

47) Shoenfeld, Y. "Vaccination and Autoimmunity-'Vaccinosis': A Dangerous Liaison?" *National Center for Biotechnology Information.* US National Library of Medicine. Web. 14 May 2012. <http://www.ncbi.nlm.nih.gov/pubmed/10648110>.

48) Stübgen, J.P. "Neuromuscular Disorders Associated with Hepatitis B Vaccination." *National Center for Biotechnology Information.* US National Library of Medicine. Web. 14 May 2012. <http://www.ncbi.nlm.nih.gov/pubmed/20207367>.

49) Stevenson, Heidi. "Vaccination Adjuvant Works by Killing Cells: Cause of Autoimmune Disorders?" Web. 14 May 2012. <http://www.gaia-health.com/articles451/000498-aluminum-adjuvant-kills-cells.shtml>.

50) "Studie Zur Gesundheit Von Kindern Und Jugendlichen in Deutschland." *Robert-Koch-Institut.* Web. 14 May 2012. <http://www.kiggs.de/service/english/index.html>.

51) *TheFreeDictionary.com.* Web. 14 May 2012. <http://medical-dictionary.thefreedictionary.com/drug>.

52) Tomljenovic, Shaw. "Do Aluminum Vaccine Adjuvants Contribute to the Rising Prevalence of Autism?" *National Center for Biotechnology Information.* US National Library of Medicine. Web. 15 May 2012. <http://www.ncbi.nlm.nih.gov/pubmed/22099159>.

53) Tomljenovic, Shaw. "Human Papillomavirus (HPV) Vaccine Policy and Evidence-based Medicine: Are They at Odds?" *National Center for Biotechnology Information.* US National Library of Medicine. Web. 15 May 2012. <http://www.ncbi.nlm.nih.gov/pubmed/22188159>.

54) Tomljenovic, Shaw L. "Mechanisms of Aluminum Adjuvant Toxicity and Autoimmunity in Pediatric Populations." *National Center for Biotechnology Information.* US National Library of Medicine. Web. 14 May 2012. <http://www.ncbi.nlm.nih.gov/pubmed/22235057>.

55) "A Tripling of Diabetes." *Shots in the Dark.* Web. 14 May 2012. <http://www.woodmed.com/index.php/shots-in-the-dark?start=4>.

56) Tyson, Peter. "The Hippocratic Oath Today." *PBS.* PBS, 27 Mar. 2001. Web. 14 May 2012. <http://www.pbs.org/wgbh/nova/body/hippocratic-oath-today.html>.

57) "Vaccine Adverse Event Reporting System." *Centers for Disease Control and Prevention.* Centers for Disease Control and Prevention, 08 Feb. 2011. Web.

14 May 2012. <http://www.cdc.gov/vaccinesafety/Activities/vaers.html>.

58) "Vaccine Injury Compensation." *Vaccine Injury Compensation*. Web. 14 May 2012. <http://www.nvic.org/injury-compensation.aspx>.

59) "Vaccine Injury Table." *Vaccine Injury Table*. Web. 14 May 2012. <http://www.hrsa.gov/vaccinecompensation/vaccinetable.html>.

60) "Vaccine Side Effects." *Vaccine Side Effects*. Web. 14 May 2012. <http://www.healingourchildren.net/vaccine_side_effects.htm>.

61) "The Vaccine Xchange." *The Vaccine Xchange*. Web. 14 May 2012. <http://vaccinexchange.org/2012/01/07/how-the-fda-plays-doctors-and-parents-for-fools-and-how-to-stop-them/>.

62) "VAERS Database." *Search VAERS Database*. Web. 14 May 2012. <http://medalerts.org/vaersdb/index.php>.

63) <http://www.uscfc.uscourts.gov/sites/default/files/MILLMAN.Werderitsh.pdf>.

64) White, Patti. "Hepatitis B Vaccine Hearings." *Patti White Testimony to Congress*. Web. 14 May 2012. <http://www.vaccinationnews.com/rally/School-NurseTestimony.htm>.

65) Wilson, K. "Adverse Events following 12 and 18 Month Vaccinations: A Population-based, Self-controlled Case Series Analysis." *National Center for*

Biotechnology Information. US National Library of Medicine. Web. 14 May 2012. <http://www.ncbi.nlm. nih.gov/pubmed/22174753>.

66) "Wirksamkeitsnachweis." *Impfkritik.de.* Web. 14 May 2012. <http://www.impfkritik.de/wirksam-keitsnachweis/>.

67) Zafrir, Z. „Autoimmunity Following Hepatitis B Vaccine as Part of the Spectrum of ; Autoimmune (Auto-inflammatory) Syndrome Induced by Adju-vants; (ASIA): Analysis of 93 Cases." *National Center for Biotechnology Information.* US National Library of Medicine. Web. 14 May 2012. <http://www.ncbi.nlm. nih.gov/pubmed/22235045>.

68) (http://www.vacinfo.org/MS-HepB.pdf).

(End Notes)

1 Tomljenovic

2 Wilson

3 Krawitt

4 Marichal

5 Stevenson

6 Mercola

7 Miller

8 Lisa

9 Tomljenovic

10 Sellers

11 Little Ben Trust

12 The Vaccine Xchange

13 Vaccine Injury Compensation

14 Vaccine Adverse Event Reporting System

15 Cynthia

16 Braun

17 Vaccine Injury Table

18 About Us

19 Adams

20 Adams

21 Adams

22 Adams

23 Adams

24 Adams

25 Rota

26 Healthsentinel.com

27 Vaccine Side Effects

28 Centers for Disease Control and Prevention

29 Colebeck

30 Immunization Science

31 Studie Zur Gesundheit Von Kindern Und Jugendlichen in Deutschland

32 Kögel-Schauz

33 Tomljenovic

34 Tomljenovic

35 Tomljenovic

36 Geier

37 Meroni

38 Karali

39 Haemophilus B Conjugate Vaccine

40 HAEMOPHILUS B CONJUGATE

41 Poliovirus Vaccine Inactivated

42 Mercola

43 Mercola

44 Mercola

45 Adams

46 VAERS Database

47 RotaTeq Oral Solution

48 RotaTeq Oral Solution

49 Doctor of Vaccine Profit

50 Blaylock

51 Wirksamkeitsnachweis

52 Tyson

53 7 Signs of a Bad Doctor

54 TheFreeDictionary.com

55 Aluminum Toxicity

56 Schneeweiss

57 Merriam-Webster

58 Tomljenovic

59 Tomljenovic

60 De Veer

61 Zafrir

62 Stübgen

63 Maya

64 Buttram

65 "Definition of 'Quack'"

66 Prevalence and Incidence of Type 1 Diabetes

67 Prevalence and Incidence of Type 1 Diabetes

68 Nakazawa

69 Shoenfeld

70 Tomljenovic

71 How Vaccines Work

72 A Tripling of Diabetes

73 Dunbar

74 Living with Diabetes

75 White

76 White

77 White

78 Belkin

79 Belkin

80 Web

81 Gran

82 Olson

83 Commenge

84 Vaccine Info

Made in the USA
San Bernardino, CA
14 September 2013